INVEST IN YOURSELF *with* EXERCISE

Tactics to Build the Exercise Habit and Enrich & Energize Your Workouts

SUSAN SMITH JONES, PhD
FOREWORD BY DAVID CRADDOCK

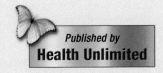

Published by
Health Unlimited

The health suggestions and recommendations in this book are based on the training, research and personal experiences of the author. Because each person and each situation is unique, the author and publisher encourage the reader to check with his or her physician or other health professional before using any procedure outlined in this book. Neither the author nor the publisher is responsible for any adverse consequences resulting from any of the suggestions in this book.

Cover and book design: Gary A. Rosenberg

Published by Health Unlimited
Los Angeles, CA

ISBN: 978-0-9991492-0-1

For further information and permission approval, contact:

Health Unlimited, PO Box 49215, Los Angeles, CA 90049, Attn. Manager

This book is lovingly dedicated to everyone who wants to . . . create vibrant, robust health and fitness; lose weight and keep it off for good; attract wealth and prosperity; experience deeper levels of joy and happiness; establish more satisfying relationships; succeed with work and career; tap into the fountain of peace within; and live a more balanced and soul-satisfying life.

I know you can do it and I applaud your courage, perseverance and commitment.

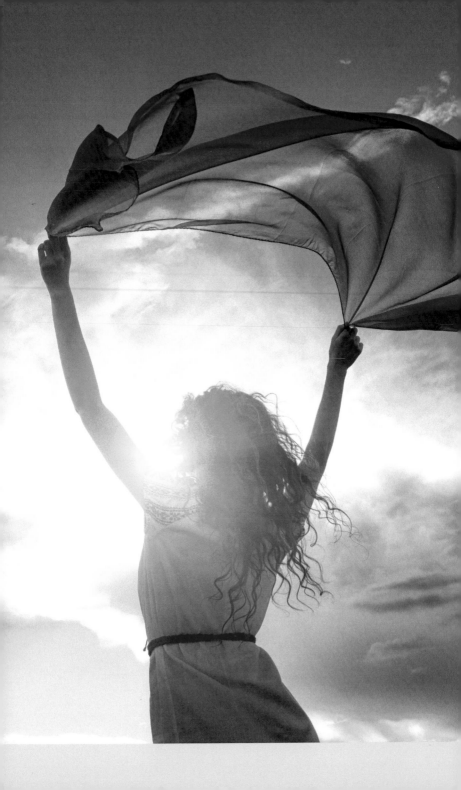

QUOTES ABOUT HEALTH & EXERCISE
FOR INSPIRATION & MOTIVATION

*Everyone's dream can come true
if you just stick to it and work hard.*
—SERENA WILLIAMS

*Her pleasure in the walk must arise
from the exercise and the day.*
—JANE AUSTEN

The first wealth is health.
—RALPH WALDO EMERSON

*Take care of your body.
It's the only place you have to live.*
—JIM ROHN

*Physical fitness is not only one of
the most important keys to a healthy
body, it is the basis of dynamic and
creative intellectual activity.*
—JOHN F. KENNEDY

*An early morning walk is a
blessing for the entire day.*

—HENRY DAVID THOREAU

*If you are seeking creative ideas,
go out walking. Angels whisper to
a man when he goes for a walk.*

—RAYMOND INMON

*If we could give every individual the right
amount of nourishment and exercise,
not too little and not too much, we would
have found the safest way to health.*

—HIPPOCRATES

*All truly great thoughts are
conceived while walking.*

—FRIEDRICH NIETZSCHE

*It is exercise alone that supports the
spirits, and keeps the mind in vigor.*

—CICERO

*The more you praise and celebrate your
life, the more there is to celebrate.*

—OPRAH WINFREY

Contents

PART 3: Set Up a Positive Magnetic Force

PART 4: Surefire Tips to Enjoy, Enrich & Energize Your Workouts

---

PART 5: How Prayer-Walking & Prayer-Hiking Can Enrich Your Life— Physically, Emotionally, Mentally & Spiritually

---

AFTERWORD: More Inspirational Quotes for Encouragement

Foreword

By David Craddock

> *Each patient carries his own*
> *doctor inside him.*
> —ALBERT SCHWEITZER

When Dr. Susan asked me if I would write the foreword for her book *Invest in Yourself with Exercise: Tactics to Build the Exercise Habit and Enrich & Energize Your Workouts,* I was delighted. For years she has been my holistic health guru and coach, teaching me how to create vibrant health and get fit and strong. As a result, I now feel about 30 years younger than I did just a few years ago, and people tell me that I look better than I have in decades. My work with Susan has given me the fountain of youth and vitality. But I'm getting ahead of myself. Let me start back at the beginning.

It was June 2009 when my health seemed to be at an all-time low. In England where I live, I focused much of my time on my career and didn't put time into my health needs. I had terrible allergies (they plagued me for 30 years) and I definitely needed to lose lots of weight. I didn't know where to turn for the holistic help I desired.

There's a saying that . . . *When the student is ready, the teacher will appear.* One day I was talking to my mum (Marjorie) about my health issues. As always, in her positive approach to life, she said to me, "You will find the answers you seek." That same day, I got in the mail some information about a 3-Day Holistic Health Conference that would be held in London featuring many world-renowned health and human potential speakers. They were all experts in their fields from around the world, but the only one that truly caught my attention was the speaker Susan Smith Jones, PhD. She was giving three presentations on all aspects of healing and rejuvenating the body, mind and spirit, and I knew at that moment that I needed to attend.

Before I got this conference information, I had already known about Susan's work. Marjorie and I had been reading many of her articles in magazines in the UK and America, we had a couple of her many books, and I saw her on a TV talk show when I was in New York City. On a few occasions, we even heard her on BBC radio talk shows in the UK and saw her on some British TV talk shows. We always enjoyed her holistic, practical and positive approach to wellness, balanced living and creating our best lives.

Marjorie and I attended the conference together in London and were not disappointed. Susan's three presentations were life-changing for us. One was about fitness and simple, practicable ways to create a strong, lean body and how to stay motivated to exercise for life. Another one of her talks was about nutrition and how to fuel the body with the healthiest foods and break unhealthy food habits. And her third presentation was all about the essential "healthy living extras," as Susan would always refer to them—the other wellness components that can make a profound difference in how we look and feel, such a sleep, water hydration, stress reduction, meditation, positive relationships, an attitude of gratitude and more.

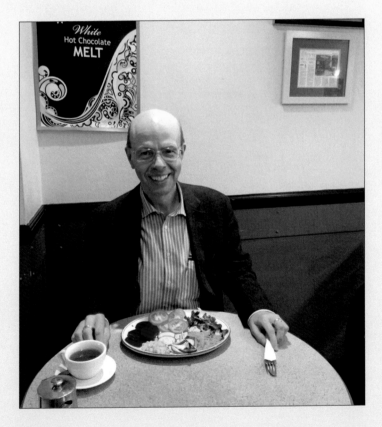

I couldn't get enough of her talks. Throughout all three, I was taking copious notes as I sat in the front row each time. During the question and answer sessions of each talk, I was always the first person to raise my hand and seek to get clarification of things she discussed. Susan was always patient, thoughtful and sensitive to my questions and other people's questions in the room. It was clear with her three standing ovations that everyone else in the room appreciated her three talks as much as I did.

At the end of the third presentation, I asked Susan if she would be willing to meet with me privately in the lecture hall after everyone left to talk about some of my health concerns and possibly even agree to work with me. During that first session with her, I knew for sure that I was guided to the best teacher for me. Susan is knowledgeable and kind, has a wonderful sense of humor and knows how to inspire, motivate and empower her clients. When I asked if she would agree to coach me on how to get healthy and fit, she agreed and suggested that I fly to Santa Monica (Los Angeles) with Marjorie the following January, 2010 to "start the year off with a positive commitment to health and youthful vitality," she said.

This trip and time with Susan turned out to be a godsend for Marjorie and me. For two weeks we stayed at a hotel on the bluff in Santa Monica and every day and evening, Susan worked with both Marjorie (she was 80) and me, teaching us about all of the principles and practices of a healthy lifestyle. I needed to lose weight and get healthy and Marjorie needed to gain weight and become mobile again. Marjorie arrived in a wheelchair, barely able to walk on her own, and I resolved to achieve significant improvement in my health and was open to any guidance Susan would be giving me.

On day one, Susan took both of us to the hotel's fully loaded gym to do weight training and use the aerobic equipment, which we did every day we were there. She took me hiking in the mountains of Santa Monica, for long walks on the beach, and taught us many other enjoyable ways to exercise that were actually pleasurable such as exercising in the swimming pool in the beautiful sunshine of Santa Monica (quite different from England's weather)! All the time, she would talk to us both with great detail about why we should or should not do things a certain way, and yes, I continued to takes loads of notes daily. Susan showed us how to order off restaurant menus for healthy selections, how to shop at grocery stores for the healthiest foods, made sure we were well-hydrated, sleep eight hours at night and she made the process of getting healthy really fun!

One of my favorite exercises in the gym is the rowing machine. Susan taught me how to row with good form to prevent injury and get the maximum benefits and now I row several times weekly. It's my favorite aerobic activity in the gym because it's great as a cardio workout, but it is also an excellent endurance- and strength-builder.

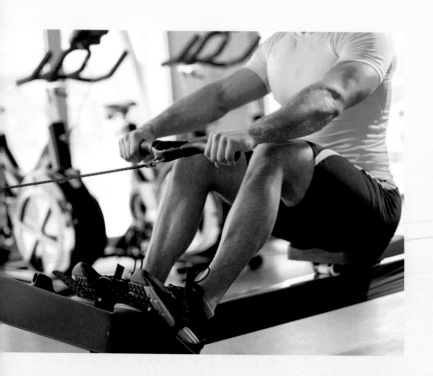

When we arrived in Los Angeles, Susan promised she would give us both her recipe for the "fountain of youth" and teach us how to maintain it when we got back home to England. Well, she did accomplish this and so much more. Marjorie arrived in Santa Monica unable to walk without assistance and 14 days later, Marjorie built up to walking three miles a day without help, and was gobsmacked at how great she felt. In fact, she didn't want to leave Susan or the sunshine. Marjorie had never stepped foot in a gym before this trip, and she grew to love the weight training because she could see her strength increasing by the day. Susan patiently helped her feel comfortable with the weights and aerobic machines and watched her every movement.

Mum was over-the-moon with joy and vitality when she left and had gained six pounds, exactly what she needed. Oh, by the way, when we got back to England, Marjorie joined our local gym and kept weight training regularly. In fact, the local newspaper in our town in England wrote an article about Marjorie and her weight training, as she was the oldest member of the gym.

When I arrived under Susan's holistic care on the first day, after weight training, I noticed how tired I felt after our one-mile jog. By the last few days, I was weight training for one hour, hiking the steep mountains in

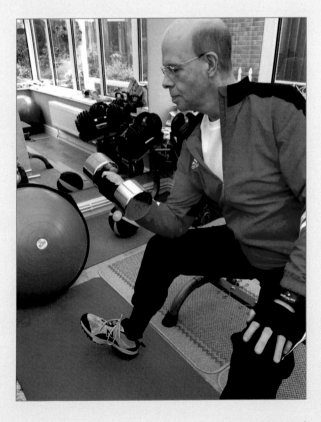

Santa Monica for three hours with Susan, and jogging on the soft sand of the beach for another workout—all in the same day! In-between these arduous workouts, we would stretch often to increase flexibility.

Susan introduced me to something called myo-fascial trigger point therapy on my body. From constantly sitting at my desk, in my car, on trains and in airplanes, without ever doing any stretching and other flexibility exercises, she said I had many palpable nodules in taut bands of muscle fibers, and these "knots" are an identifiable source of pain in my muscles and

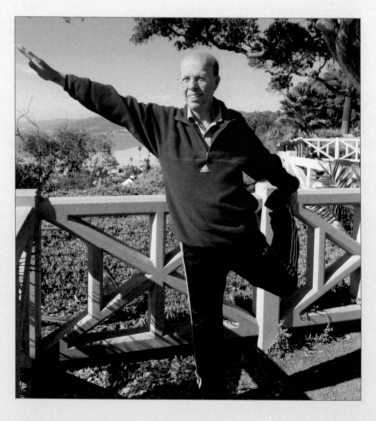

were affecting so many areas of my body, including my posture. After only three sessions with Susan on my many trigger points, I no longer felt any pain in my back and shoulders that I had been experiencing for a few years.

Another one of her promises to me was that if I would follow her allergy program for four months when I got home, I would be rid of my allergies for good after 30 years of this annoyance. She was right. Within just under four months of taking some nutritional supplements and cleaning up my diet, keeping more hydrated and getting more sleep, my allergies were gone and have never returned.

I returned back to England 13 pounds lighter in 14 days, and we ate all day long. It was like a miracle to me! I learned a whole new way of eating—choosing delicious high fiber, nutrient-rich foods. Those two weeks under Susan's guidance changed my health and life for the better. Since my visit with Susan in 2010, I've continued with her healthy living program, have lost a total of 75 pounds through regular exercise and a healthy diet, and she checks in with me regularly to fine-tune my personal plan of action for optimum health and youthful vitality . . . always. I can honestly say that I have never felt better in my life than I do right now.

Presently, I eat a clean, healthy, lean diet and choose organic foods, whenever possible. It's easy to order at restaurants now because most menus have healthy alternatives or the chefs are willing and happy to prepare healthy dishes for me.

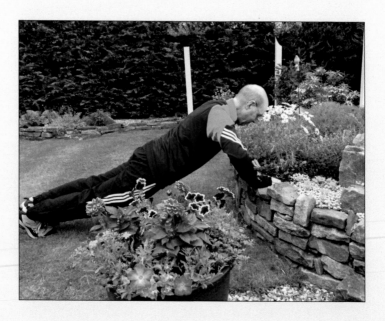

Because of Susan's positive teachings, combined with my desire to stay healthy, happy, strong and fit well into older age, I now usually workout in the local gym in town four to six days weekly. Susan even came over and helped me set up a home gym with some aerobic equipment (yes it includes a rowing machine), a couple benches, dumbbells and other machines. This way when my schedule is really tight with work, conferences and meetings, I still have a place in my home to exercise. And now, when I travel to locations around the world to give my lectures and presentations and to meet with clients, I always take my fitness clothes to get in power walks or jogs; I find hotels that have in-house gyms; and I pack in my luggage exercise bands which weigh next to nothing that are simple to use in the hotel room.

In all her sagacity, Susan always reminded me that . . . "When you commit to something like an exercise program, don't let your excuses get in your way. You must follow through on your commitment to fitness and arrange your personal circumstances so that your lifestyle totally supports your commitment." She'd often tell me to . . . "Do the things you need to do to order your life, eliminate non-essentials and focus on what is important."

Susan helped me to understand that if we don't have health, we lose our enjoyment and appreciation of life. It is truly our greatest wealth. She taught me that I am the president and CEO of my body and life and it's up to me to take great care of my body. Here's something she emphasized often to me: "To become master of your outer life, you must first become master of your inner world—CEO of your mind. Teach your mind how to think differently: how to be calm, loving, courageous and optimistic. The body reflects the mind and the mind reflect the spirit; all three are connected and holistic health incorporates the loving care of the whole person. Eating healthy foods gives you a more positive attitude. Choosing to be grateful for your miraculous body makes it easier to exercise and get ample sleep at night. So each day make your health a top priority and take loving care of your body with nutritious foods, daily exercise, positive living habits and a cheerful attitude." I will never forget her teachings and now in my work with other people, I will often share with them some of the health- and life-enriching teachings I learned from Susan.

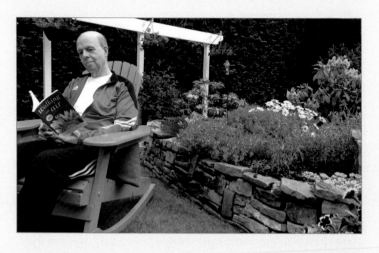

So when she asked me if I would write this foreword for her book, it was my great pleasure. In the pages of this informative and uplifting book, you'll learn from Susan the importance of exercise for overall high-level wellness; how to get the most from your workouts; ways to stay motivated to exercise; tips to prevent exercise boredom, burnout and injury; the best exercises to look younger, bolster energy and lose weight; how to fight excess fat by mastering your metabolism; how to incorporate prayer-walking to enhance mental and spiritual health; ways to turn dreams into reality; the power of choice; and much more.

"An investment in yourself and in your health," as Susan repeated to me often in our training and teaching sessions, "is the best investment you can make." This book will inspire, motivate and empower you, too.

David Craddock, MA (Oxon), BA (Hons)
www.DavidCraddock.com
www.TimeForInvestment.com

*Far away there in the sunshine are
my highest aspirations. I may not
reach them, but I can look at them
to see their beauty, believe in them,
and try to follow where they lead.*

—Louisa May Alcott

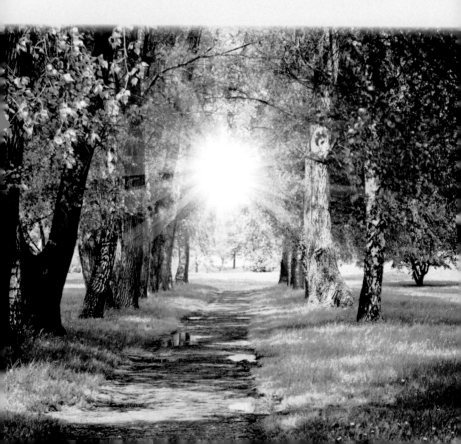

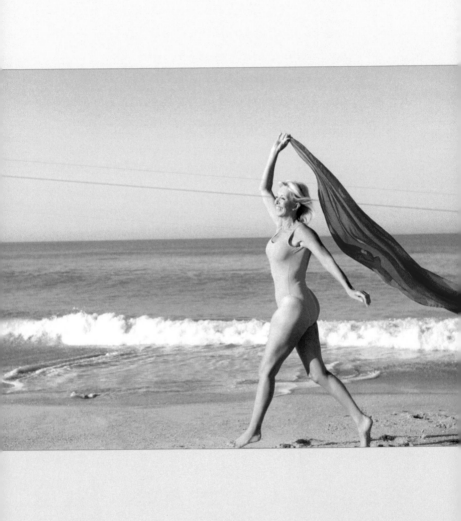

PART 1

Using Exercise as Medicine

> *I still get wildly enthusiastic*
> *about little things . . . I play with*
> *leaves. I skip down the street,*
> *and run against the wind.*
>
> —LEO BUSCAGLIA

Hello Friend,

IT IS WITH GREAT JOY THAT I AM WRITING THIS BOOK for you. My hope is that it will inspire, motivate and empower you to make regular exercise a part of your daily lifestyle. Exercise is the key to youthful vitality . . . at any age. It unlocks brainpower, physical stamina and mental clarity. It gives your skin a youthful glow and puts wings under your confidence. I'll go so far to say that nothing does more to make you vibrantly healthy than a regular fitness program. By the time you reach the end of this book, my wish is that you'll be so encouraged that you will immediately start exercising in some way, and from that day forward, make exercise a non-negotiable part of your new, healthy and vigorous lifestyle.

We all know exercise is a key component of vibrant health. Yet statistics reveal that only about 25% of people in the USA and the UK make exercise a regular part of their lifestyle. My hope is that after reading this book, if you're not already a fitness enthusiast, you'll be helping to increase the percentage. Whether you have several children and are busy with them from morning to night, or are CEO of a Fortune 500 company or international conglomerate and put in 12–16 hours a day seven days a week at the job, or you are retired and not very active at all, you must find time to exercise.

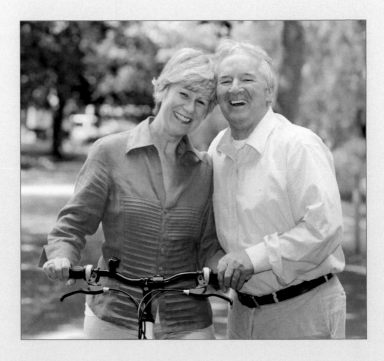

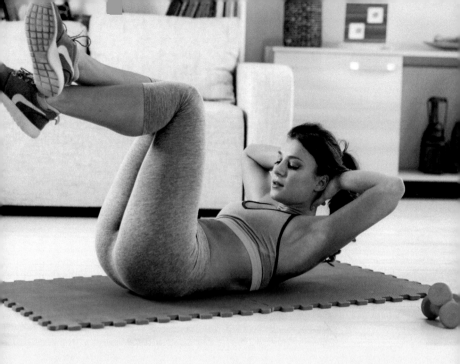

If you can't carve out an hour a day to exercise, or even thirty minutes, then break the time up into 10- or 15-minute allotments. I don't believe in gimmicks and potions and magic pills, and I promise you there is no substitute for exercise. The old "I don't have time to exercise" excuse just doesn't work with me. You must make fitness a priority—a nonnegotiable part of your day.

You need—we all need—to find some type of physical activity that fits into your lifestyle and that exercises not only your body but also your mind and spirit. If there is one self-help idea that has really caught on and that I'm sure will stay with us, it's the idea that physical fitness transcends the physical body to benefit your mental and spiritual fitness as well.

Staying Motivated to Exercise

Kim used to do all her workouts in the gym. Four to five mornings a week, before dawn, she went to her gym and walked on the treadmill, staring out into space, oblivious to her immediate environment. I saw her for weeks doing the same 45 minutes on the treadmill, only occasionally switching to the bike or the elliptical machine. Then one day I introduced myself after her workout was complete and told her I had just finished my strength training routine. I asked her about her workout. She admitted to me that although what she did was convenient and gave her good results, it was boring. "I am a morning person, so it's not too hard getting up before the rest of the world," she said to me, "but it's often hard to motivate myself to get on the treadmill and do the same old thing."

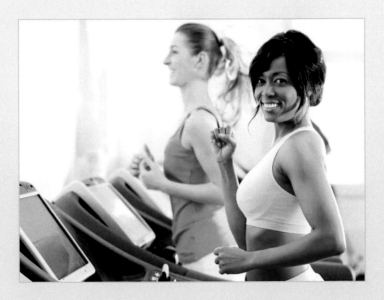

Then she asked what I liked to do for my cardio training, so I told her about my passion for hiking and being outdoors, whenever possible, to workout. "There's something about being in nature, feeling the sun, breathing the fresh air, absorbing the mood-lifting negative ions and actually going somewhere, as opposed to walking in place, that makes the time fly and makes the workout fun," I told Kim. She was intrigued, and I asked her if she would like to accompany me on a hike the following morning.

We agreed to meet at the head of one of the Santa Monica (in Los Angeles) hiking trails, just minutes from both of our homes, at the same time she usually works out, six in the morning. Her experience was no different from that of my many other friends and clients who started in the gym and are now avid hikers. I shared with Kim about my experiences hiking in the United Kingdom (UK) and around the world.

When hiking you can take in a variety of terrain, flora and fauna while soaking up a wide range of sensations, sights, sounds and scents as you move and work out your entire body. Hiking strengthens your body and feeds your soul, in other words, and you feel invigorated throughout the day. Of course, seasonal and weather changes offer further variety as your program continues throughout the year, as does an occasional change of location. For three decades I've told my clients and friends that making exercise fun should be as high a priority as making it effective. And even if you don't live in a climate that's conducive to exercising outdoors

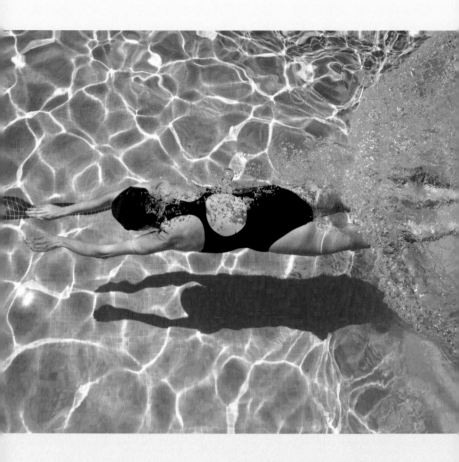

year-round, you can still add fun into workouts simply by listening to terrific music, going to a gym that motivates you, watching an exercise DVD that's invigorating or simply parking at the end of a parking lot when out and about and walking faster to your location. I do this frequently when I travel and still want to get in some exercise. Lightweight and easily packed exercise bands and an upbeat music CD can do wonders for exercising in a hotel room.

How to Use Exercise as Medicine and a Natural Healer

Patterns of modern living have channeled the average American into an increasingly sedentary existence. We human beings, however, were designed and built for movement, and our bodies have not adapted well to this reduced level of activity.

For many adults with sedentary occupations, physical activity provides an outlet for job-related tensions or mental fatigue. In addition to reducing tension in the body, exercise can boost spirits and help us feel good about ourselves. Exercise has also been found to aid in weight control or reduction, to improve posture and to increase energy. Further, my research and experience indicates that many cases, in fact 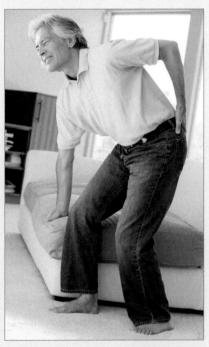 about half of lower back pain can be traced to poor abdominal muscle tone and back inflexibility. Proper exercise can often prevent or correct lower back pain. Research also indicates that much of the degeneration of bodily function and structure associated with pre-mature aging seems to be reduced by a program of vigorous, regular exercise.

Regular exercise is necessary then to develop and maintain not only an optimal level of health, but also a youthful appearance, mental clarity and high energy. Regular exercise increases muscle strength and endurance. It enhances the function of the lungs, heart and blood vessels; increases the flexibility of the joints; and improves coordination and efficiency of movement.

It is easy to see why the case for exercise is so strong. What's not so easy is implementing it in your life and sticking to it, and in Part 3 of this book, I will give you surefire tips to stay motivated to exercise and to prevent exercise boredom, burnout and injury.

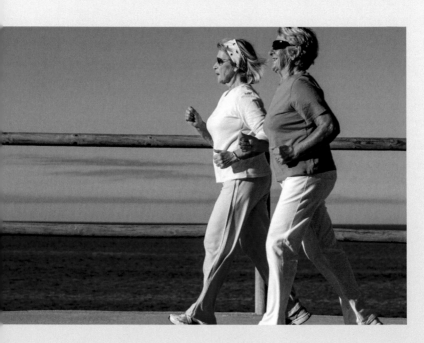

More Reasons to Exercise
for Health Enhancement

But before you can experience any of the benefits of vigorous exercise, you must take responsibility for your own fitness program and for choosing those activities that promote fitness. My aim in this section of the book is to cite research that will convince you of the advantages of following a well-rounded fitness program. I will concentrate on how exercise contributes to your self-image, happiness and peace of mind. I have gone into this topic in much greater detail in my books, *Living on the Lighter Side*, *The Joy Factor*, *Walking on Air* and *Healthy, Happy & Radiant . . . at Any Age*. There you'll find loads more information that will empower you to make exercise a regular part of your health program.

"A sound mind in a sound body" is a traditional Latin motto. Researchers are finding, however, that there's much more to the adage than might first appear. It seems that our sense of happiness and well-being depends on how much exercise we get. Malcolm Carruthers, head of a British medical team, believes that "most people could ban the blues with a simple, vigorous 10-minute exercise session three times a week." He came to this conclusion after spending four years studying the effect of norepinephrine on 200 people. Norepinephrine is a depression-destroying hormone, "The chemical key to happiness," according to Carruthers. Ten minutes of exercise doubles the level of norepinephrine in the body.

Enkephalin is another spirit-lifting chemical produced in the brain during vigorous aerobic exercise. Enkephalins are the source of the feeling known as runner's high among the long-distance runners that have been studied often. Enkephalin is a type of endorphin, morphine-like chemicals that serve as natural opiates, increasing pain tolerance and producing euphoric feelings. A study at Massachusetts General Hospital found a rise of more than 145 percent in endorphins during one hour of vigorous exercise. So you might want to honor the words I tell all of my clients: "Walk your dog every day, whether you have a dog or not."

Exercise can work in conjunction with psychotherapy to alleviate depression, according to work done at

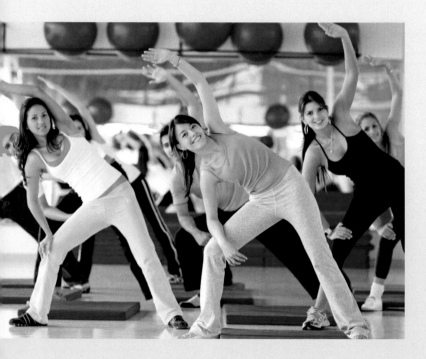

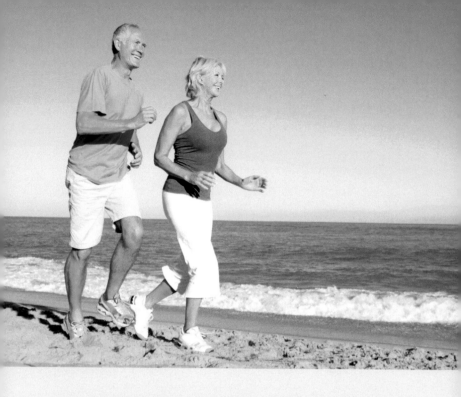

the Menninger Clinic in Topeka, Kansas. "It's not a panacea, but it is a useful adjunct for treating depression," says the clinic's Robert Conroy. One of Conroy's hypotheses is that exercise boosts self-image by changing an individual's worldview from that of passive bystander to active participant. People who exercise believe they have control over their health and the quality of their lives.

Exercise works better than tranquilizers to eliminate symptoms of tension and anxiety. Herbert de Vries, former exercise physiology lab director at the University of Southern California, conducted a classic study of tense and anxious people. As one part of the experiment, he administered 400-milligram doses of meprobamate, the main ingredient in many tranquil-izers. In the second part, he had the same group of people take a walk vigorous enough to raise their heart rates over 100 beats per minute. De Vries measured tension levels by monitoring the amount of electrical activity in the subjects' muscles. "Measuring electrical activity in muscles is the most objective way to mea-sure a person's nervousness," he says. He found that after exercise, electrical activity was 20 percent less than the subjects' normal rate. After being dosed with meprobamate, the subjects showed little change in the electrical activity in their muscles. "Movement is strong medicine," de Vries concluded.

By releasing tension, exercise also leads to a good night's sleep, a key to mental well-being. Martin Cohn,

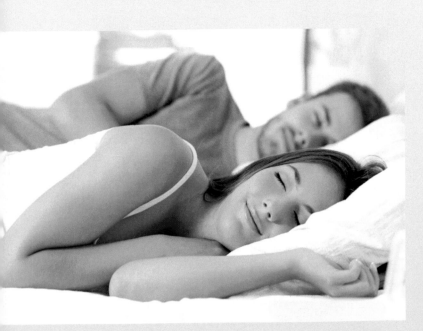

MD, chief of the Sleep Disorders Clinic at Sinai Hospital in Miami, agrees. "Exercise helps you deal with tension and provides a healthy release," he says. "And this is the key to a good night's sleep, a necessary component of mental well-being." You know how well you sleep if you've been walking regularly or going to the gym.

One of the body's nonspecific responses to stress is to release catecholamine, a substance related to epinephrine. It has been found that exercise not only reduces nervous anxiety but also reduces the amount of catecholamines.

"Chronic tension states," say Dr. Paul Insel and Dr. Walton Roth of the Stanford University Medical Center, "are known to be associated with numerous bodily malfunctions such as ulcers, migraine headaches, asthma, skin eruptions, high blood pressure and even heart disease." Psychological symptoms include irritability, touchiness, moodiness and depression. "Running," the doctors say, "has been shown to relieve some of these symptoms. It does this by pulling the plug on pent-up tension."

Dr. William P. Morgan of the University of Wisconsin tested the lactate theory — the idea that exercise negatively alters the body's chemical balance, thus making it tenser. He found that lactate released by exercise differed significantly from the chemical substance that had been injected into anxious patients, and that exercise-induced chemical changes led to a "definite decrease in anxiety levels in normal and neurotic individuals."

Create a Well-Rounded Fitness Program

Most researchers point to the need for a combination of weight training and aerobic activity to produce truly beneficial psychological and biochemical changes. This is also true for cardiovascular improvements. This is why the emphasis is placed on weight training, jogging, brisk walking, swimming, cycling and other forms of aerobics. These vigorous, rhythmic activities appear to send messages to the brain as well as the endocrine system to shape up and feel good.

Of course, to any well-rounded program, you must also add in exercises that promote flexibility such at yoga, Pilates or just simple stretching. As a former fitness instructor to students, staff and faculty at the University of California, Los Angeles (UCLA) for 30 years, and the first fitness trainer in Los Angeles in the

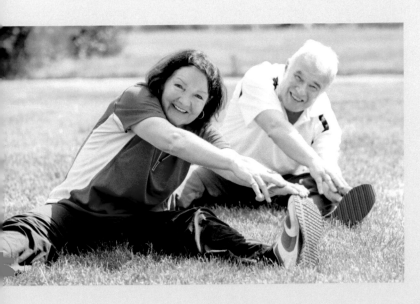

'70s, I know the importance of keeping the muscles, ligaments, tendons and connective tissue flexible. In order to do this, you must engage in flexibility exercises at least three times a week. I feel best when I do my stretching routine six times a week. The older you get, the tighter your entire body becomes.

Additionally, I recommend doing some work with myofascial trigger points, known as trigger points. On a regular basis, I see a bodyworker to release my muscular trigger points (to work out my "knots") to improve motion in my spine and entire body, which helps the brain and nervous system. I always feel happier and more relaxed and peaceful after my sessions. Trigger point release work restores proper muscular function and neurologic function to all of the organs in the body. It's effective in assuaging pain in the back, neck, knees, hips, shoulders, hands and wrists, feet, legs, groin and more, as well as for headaches. It is even helpful for chest tightness. I encourage you to find someone in your area who specializes in trigger point therapy—look for a chiropractor, physical therapist, osteopathic practitioner, massage therapist or a shiatsu specialist who knows about trigger point work.

How often are we presented with a means to take control of our psychological and physical well-being through something as enjoyable and rewarding as exercise? The message is clear. A well-designed fitness program can add years of fulfilling, vibrant health. And that knowledge alone has a potent positive effect on mental well-being.

> Health is a complete package: physical, mental and spiritual. Show by your daily actions that health is a top priority for you. With a positive mindset, you can accomplish anything.

HUMOR  TIME

Between the parts of this book, I have created four Humor Time breaks with some funny jokes or phrases about exercise, weight loss and health in general. Everybody loves to laugh. In fact, did you know that laughter is very good for you? It was Norman Cousin who said: "Laughter is a form of internal jogging." Humor and laughter have both been found to be important components of healing. It's been reported that laughter aids digestion, stimulates the heart, strengthens muscles, activates the brain's creative function and keeps you alert. Laughter also helps you to keep things in better perspective. So make up your mind to laugh and to be happy. When you laugh at yourself, you take yourself far less seriously. "Angels fly because they take themselves lightly," says an old Scottish proverb. Isn't that wonderful?

I simply love to laugh and am known to be a practical joker! My mother June called laughter "the body's elixir" or natural rejuvenator. It is an essential ingredient to daily living and something I use to fuel my spirituality. Because of my positive, easygoing, "lighten up" approach to life, I have acquired the nickname "Sunny" because I am always reminding others to not take life so seriously.

So let's start with this first batch of jokes and funny phrases.

*In two decades I've lost a total of
789 pounds. I should be hanging
from a charm bracelet.*

—Erma Bombeck

*It is well documented that for every
mile that you jog, you add one minute
to your life. This enables you at 85 years
old to spend an additional 5 months in
a nursing home at $5,000 per month.*

—Unknown

*My grandmother started walking
five miles a day when she was 60.
She's 97 now and we don't know
where the heck she is.*

—Ellen DeGeneres

*I like long walks, especially when they
are taken by people who annoy me.*

—Sir Noël Coward

*I don't exercise at all. If God meant
us to touch our toes, he would have
put them further up on our body.*

—Unknown

*I decided to take an aerobics class. I
bent . . . twisted . . . gyrated . . . jumped
up and down . . . and perspired for
a half an hour. But by the time I got
my tights on . . . the class was over!*

—UNKNOWN

*I have to exercise in the morning before
my brain figures out what I'm doing.*

—UNKNOWN

*I joined a health club last year, spent
about $400 bucks. Haven't lost a pound.
Apparently you have to show up.*

—UNKNOWN

*I have flabby thighs, but fortunately
my stomach covers them.*

—JOAN RIVERS

*God must love calories.
He made so many.*

—UNKNOWN

*The advantage of exercising every
day is that you die healthier.*

—UNKNOWN

PART 2

Fighting Excess Fat by Mastering Your Metabolism

When people tell me they can't afford to join a gym, I tell them to go outside; planet Earth is a gym and we're already members. Run, climb, sweat and enjoy all of the natural wonder that is available to you.

—Steve Mariboli

WHILE MILLIONS OF PEOPLE STARVE TO DEATH IN many parts of the world, the United States has the dubious honor of being the fattest country on the globe, with 50% of us being obese. Meanwhile, we Americans are preoccupied with our waistlines. We spend more than 40 billion dollars a year on diet foods, diet programs, diet pills and other "guaranteed" weight-loss regimens and products. Yet, according to the National Center of Health Statistics, we're getting fatter all the time.

Experts call obesity an American epidemic—one that brings with it major health problems. Heart dis-

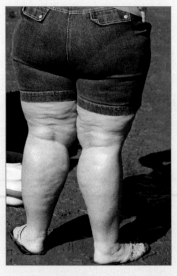

ease, endometrial (uterine) cancer and possibly breast cancer, high cholesterol, high blood pressure, immune dysfunction, osteoarthritis, stroke, gout, sleep disorders, gallstones and diabetes are all associated with obesity. Put in a more positive way, *losing even a little weight may significantly improve your health and well-being.*

On the flipside, eating disorders such as anorexia and bulimia are rampant, and women's magazines are not helping when they continue to use models who look like waifs. Take Barbie™, a doll that's part of most little girls' upbringing. This model of good looks and perfect body is giving the wrong message about what a healthy woman's body should look like. Were Barbie an actual person, her body fat would be so low that she probably wouldn't even be able to menstruate. As little girls treasure Barbie, and teens try to emulate her, she has one accessory that is consistently missing—food.

Surveys indicate that most people are not happy with their weight or the shape of their body. Half of the women and a quarter of the men in this country are currently trying to lose weight and reshape their bodies. The sad thing is that a majority of these people are going about it in the wrong way, the hard way—by dieting, which doesn't work! Throw away diet books that tell you that you can lose weight and keep it off without moving a muscle. They're rip-offs. Dieting is not the cure for excess fat. After you finish a diet, you may have lost some fat, but you have not lost your *tendency to get fat*.

Metabolism Tune-Up

The control mechanism for obesity is not diet; it's muscle metabolism. Your basal metabolic rate is the rate at which your body utilizes energy. Put another way, it has to do with how efficiently you body burns calories. Calories are the measuring unit of heat energy. When metabolism is higher, you burn more fat and

have an easier time losing weight (fat) or maintaining your ideal body weight. You can feed your muscles the best food and vitamin supplements in the world, but if they're not tuned up—if they're not exercised—they won't burn up the calories in those foods. As you age, if you don't continue to keep your muscles exercised, your metabolism slows down and

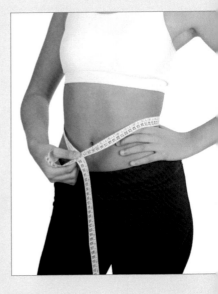

you'll gain weight more easily than you did when you were young. *Exercise is the key to controlling metabolism.*

Two out of three people who go on a diet will regain their weight in one year or less; 97% will gain the weight back in five years. To make matters worse, a majority of dieters who lose weight will gain back even more fat than they had before they started the diet. They have all violated an important rule in creating and maintaining a healthy, fast metabolism: they lost lean body mass, or muscle. An overweight person needs to retrain his or her body so that it burns up *all* the calories it gets, storing none as fat. Yes, she may need a diet at the start to help break bad eating habits, retrain her taste buds, jump-start her metabolism and lose some

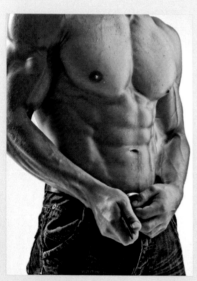

excess fat. But long-term weight control requires a change in body chemistry so you won't get fat all over again. And *exercise* is the only way to change your metabolism so that your body converts fewer calories to fat. You need aerobic exercise to burn the fat out of your muscles and then add weight training (also known as strength or resistance training) to build up your muscle, which, in turn, increases metabolism.

Your goal should be to increase your muscle mass.

Muscle burns fat. It's that simple. Exercise increases muscle, tones it, alters its chemistry, and increases the metabolic rate. When you exercise, you actually

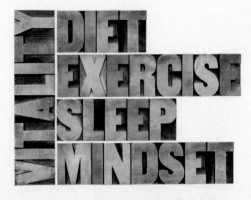

continue to burn calories even when you're sleeping but you must exercise correctly to get the best results. Before I describe the best exercises to lose fat and increase metabolism, let's briefly explore why lean muscle tissue is so important.

More muscle means a faster metabolism because muscle uses more energy to exist than fat. Because muscle is a highly metabolic tissue, it burns five times as many calories as most other body tissues, pound for pound. In other words, muscle requires more oxygen and more calories to sustain it than does body fat. When you have more muscle mass, you burn more calories than someone who doesn't, even when you're both sitting still, which is why people who build muscle have an easier time maintaining a healthy weight. They're simply more efficient calorie burners.

Following are 10 tips for increasing your metabolism, selecting efficacious exercise, choosing fat-burning foods, and making healthy choices for creating a fit, healthy body. I've used all of these guidelines with my clients worldwide over the past three decades.

1 **Increase your muscle mass.** If you increase muscle mass, you increase the number of calories your body is using every moment of the day, not just during exercise, but also at work, play, and even 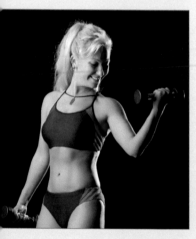 when sleeping. The addition of 10 pounds of muscle to your body will burn approximately 500 extra calories per day. You would have to jog six miles a day, seven days a week to burn the same number of calories. Ten extra pounds of muscle can burn a pound of fat in one week—that's 52 pounds of fat a year!

To increase muscle, you must engage in weight training activities. You can do these at a gym or even in the comfort of your home. Actually, it's not the weightlifting itself, but the physiological effects that take place in the 48 yours *after* weightlifting during the recovery period, that enhance metabolism. In other words, very little fat is burned during the weightlifting sessions. But *lots* of fat is burned during the recovery from weightlifting.

Well after you've finished your weight training session and you shower and are feeling refreshed and relaxed, your fat-burning enzymes are working harder than ever to repair the damage. They must replace the sugar that was used by the sugar-burning enzymes. To build up the sugar supplies (glycogen is stored muscle sugar that's used up during weightlifting), our bodies burn fat. It takes a lot of energy to restore sugar, which means that lots of calories are burned. All of this energy must be supplied by the fat-burning enzymes. That's why you must make weight training a part of your fat loss/vitality program. *Weight training stimulates metabolism and fat-burning.*

As mentioned, the best way to increase lean muscle mass is through resistance training, which means weightlifting or resistance machines—barbells, dumbbells or machines, cables or even 'free-hand' movements such as push-ups, sit-ups (crunches) and dips. All it takes to add 10 pounds of muscle is a regular weight-training program involving only 30 to 40 minutes, three times a week for about five to six months.

2 **Increase your aerobic exercise.** Aerobic exercise trains muscles to burn fat and increase metabolism. Aerobic exercise means exercising with oxygen, not being winded or out of breath. These types of exercises, which are fairly gentle and nonstop, change your metabolism and also train your muscles to burn more fat. Here's a key point to keep in mind. *Muscles burn fat only in the presence of oxygen.* For example, if you're jogging with your husband and he's breezing along and singing a song, and you're so out of breath that you can

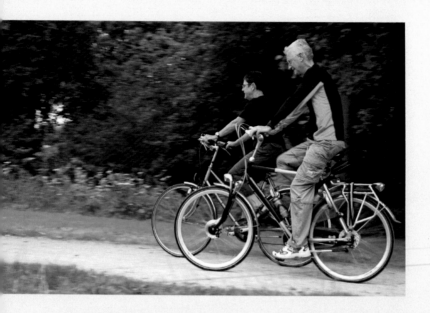

barely put two syllables together, he's burning fat but your fat-burning mechanisms have shut down. Muscles burn two kinds of fuel—sugar (glucose) and fat. Your muscles really do prefer to burn fat because it's more efficient; there's more of it so it lasts a long time and it produces lots of energy.

Does that mean you shouldn't do high-intensity sprints every so often? No, as I'll explain in tip #3, but you must make aerobic exercise part of your fitness program at least five days a week if you want to lose fat and tone up. By using the big muscles of the thighs and buttocks in an activity that is steady and nonstop (such as cross-country skiing, bicycling, rowing, walking, jogging and hiking), and makes you breathe deeply but doesn't make you out of breath, you're supplying oxygen to the muscles, which promotes fat burning in the muscles and makes you burn more food calories.

3 **Add higher intensity bursts to your exercise plan.** I work in some high-intensity activity a few times each week. For example, if I'm hiking, I'll spend 30 to 90 seconds going faster than normal on a steeper hill interspersed with more level or declining grades. (Notice I didn't say "a breakneck run." Just go a little faster than usual.) If you're cycling, pedal faster for several seconds. High intensity bursts of exercise help burn fat. Why? When you force your body to raise the level of intensity for a short burst of "getting winded," you are forcing your body to recover under stress; in other words, while you continue to exercise. This little sprint adds intensity without causing injury. And those fat-burning enzymes are realizing that not only do they need to grow when you're doing regular aerobic activity, but now they must grow even faster. In other words, *a few moments of exercising just a little bit harder than usual will help force you to recover while still exercising, which will burn more fat.* If you're just a beginner and have never exercised before, wait for about two to three weeks before add-

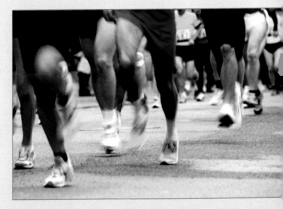

ing in these bursts of higher intensity workout and then pump up the vigor, if your doctor says you can.

4 Graze. Liquid meals, fasting and special diet packaged food aren't your answer to increasing metabolism, weight control or better health. Instead, and in addition to regular exercise, learn how to eat so that your body becomes an efficient fat-burning machine.

The results of four national surveys show that most people try to lose weight by eating 1,000 to 1,500 calories a day. However, cutting calories to under 1,200 (if you're a woman) or 1,400 (if you're a man) doesn't provide enough food to be satisfying in the long term. Eating fewer than 1,200 calories slows down metabolism and makes it difficult to get adequate amounts of certain nutrients, such as magnesium and zinc.

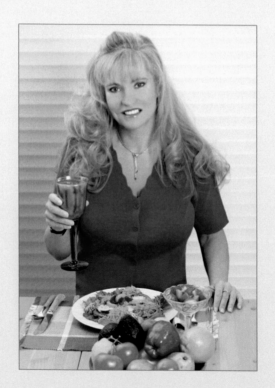

The typical dieter will often skip meals and, as research points out, the worst meal to skip, if you want to increase your metabolism, is breakfast. The word 'breakfast' means breaking a fast. This temporary fast-ing state sends a signal to the body that food is scarce. As a result, the stress hormones (including corti-sol) increase and the body begins 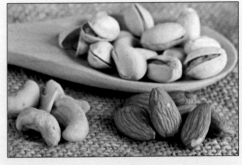 'lightening the load' and shedding its muscle tissue. Decreasing muscle tissue, as you know now is very metabolically active, decreases the body's need for food. By the next feeding, the pancreas is sensitized and will sharply increase blood insulin levels, which is the body's signal to make fat. And if you're insulin resistant, as many sedentary people are, you make extra amounts of this hormone (insulin) and make/deposit fat very easily, especially if you eat refined carbohydrates. Have you ever wondered how the Sumo wrestlers get so big? They fast and then gorge themselves with food. Clearly, this approach is absolutely counterproductive if your goal is to lose fat.

If you want to increase your metabolism, it's best to eat several small, healthy meals a day. This kind of grazing approach to meals keeps your metabolism stoked. It also keeps you from feeling deprived—a chief complaint of everyone who has ever been on a diet. As well, emphasize lots of raw foods such as fresh fruits and vegetables because these gems of nature are usually low calorie, nutrient-rich foods that support weight loss. To learn about specific foods to eat to accelerate fat loss and create a healthy, fit body, please refer to my series of three nutrition and recipe books published by Hay House comprised of *Recipes for Health Bliss, The Healing Power of NatureFoods* and *Health Bliss.*

5 **Drink lots of water daily.** Water is very important in helping to maintain a healthy metabolic rate and a fit body. Drinking at least two quarts a day, between meals, is essential—more if you're physically very active—that's about eight glasses of water daily. Water suppresses your appetite naturally. Have a large glass of water about 15 to 20 minutes before each meal or snack. I cannot stress enough how simply drinking

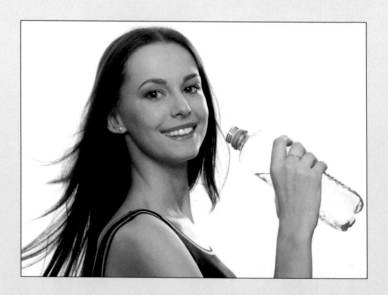

purified water—between 8 and 10 glasses of water a day—contributes greatly to fat loss and reshaping the body, even if you don't change any of your other habits.

The liver's main functions are detoxification and regulation of metabolism. The kidneys can get rid of toxins and spare the liver if they have sufficient water. This allows the liver to metabolize more fat. Adequate water will also decrease bloating and edema caused by fluid accumulation by flushing out sodium, acidic wastes and other toxins.

6 **Start your day in a positive way.** The first 40 minutes of the day always sets the tone for your entire day. So start your day in the most positive way possible. Studies show that mental and emotional stress can damage your hormonal balance—increasing your risk for weight gain. One of the best ways to reduce stress, on a daily basis, is to start your day with an enjoyable (uplifting) activity. Set aside time first thing in the morning for some light stretching, exercise, deep breathing or meditation. Make those first day-enhancing minutes healthy, positive and balanced. Another great tip would be to set 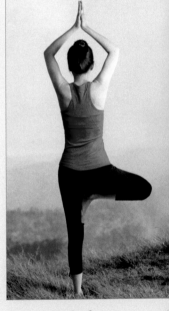 up some of your morning activities the night before. For example, lay out your exercise or work clothes, set the breakfast table, or pack healthy lunches for the day for yourself or your children to make your morning less harried and stressful. Most mornings, I sing these four lines from song *Oh, What A Beautiful Morning* from the wonderful musical *Oklahoma*. You can't sing these words and not feel happy. Here are the words . . .

> *Oh, what a beautiful mornin'*
> *Oh, what a beautiful day.*
> *I've got a beautiful feelin'*
> *Everything's goin' my way.*

7 **Avoid processed (low quality) carbohydrates and fill in with nutritional supplements.** Poor quality breads, donuts, crackers, pretzels and chips are loaded with simple sugars, genetically modified organisms (GMOs) and unhealthy fats—which increase your risk for food cravings and weight

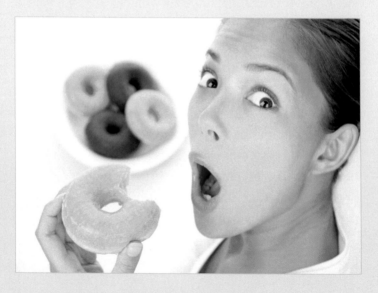

gain. What you eat, you eventually crave. Eat poor quality foods and you'll want more of them. Choose to eat colorful, healthy foods—as close to the way nature made them as possi-ble—and you'll desire more of the same. In nature, we don't find ice cream tress, donut vines, or potato chip bushes. Here's a good way to think about nutritious food:

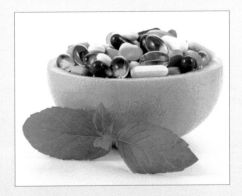

Produce is the most important health care your money can buy. Plant-based foods are rich in health-enhanc-ing fiber. Fiber-rich foods help to detoxify the digestive tract and the entire body and reduce the risk of chronic disease. Eating lots of vegetables and some fruit each day will keep you feeling 'full' and satisfied through-out the day. For example, a large salad with arugula (rocket), cucumbers, carrots, tomatoes, chickpeas, avo-cado and your favorite raw (not roasted and salted) nuts or seeds can go a long way toward nourishing the body and keeping you away from unwanted junk food.

It's always wise to take some quality nutritional supplements as insurance to help fill in any gaps where nutrients might be missing in your diet. If you visit my website, **www.SusanSmithJones.com**, and in the Search Bar put *Susan's Favorite Nutritional Supple-ments,* you will find a variety of products that I take daily and highly recommend.

8 Chew your food well and eat slowly . . .but not too slowly.

Better chewing will greatly improve digestion and actually improve your energy throughout the day. You'll probably notice that you can eat less and not feel hungry when you eat slower at mealtime. Strive to chew each bite between 15 and 30 times before swallowing.

Hormones signal the brain when you're full, but it takes about 20 minutes from start time before you feel it. Slow eating not only aids in digestion but also gives 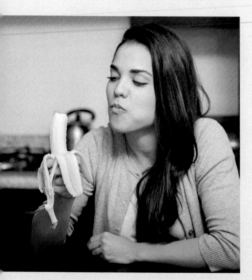 your brain a chance to know what the stomach is doing. If you make the meal last, by talking, putting down your fork between bites or just plain waiting, you're less likely to eat on "automatic pilot" and more likely to realize you're full. Combining slow eating and chewing well are essential for having control over how much you eat. You'll be amazed how much will power you can generate when you take your time and give your "satiety center" an opportunity to tell you that you aren't that hungry anymore.

On the flipside, finish your really big meals (such as holiday meals at Thanksgiving and Christmas and birthday celebrations) within an hour of starting. The body produces a second insulin hit if it senses a lot of food coming in continuously. You can avoid that second hit (and the subsequent fat storage that it triggers) by finishing within an hour of starting. If you see something you like that you forgot to eat within the hour, that's fine; just save it for tomorrow or later. It will still be there, and you won't be wearing it on your hips.

9 Get good sleep. Researchers at Columbia University in New York City found that people who slept six hours a night were 23 percent more likely to be obese than people who slept between seven and nine hours. Those who slept five hours were 50 percent more likely—while those who slept four hours or less were 73 percent more likely to be obese. Similarly, research shows that skimping on sleep interferes with

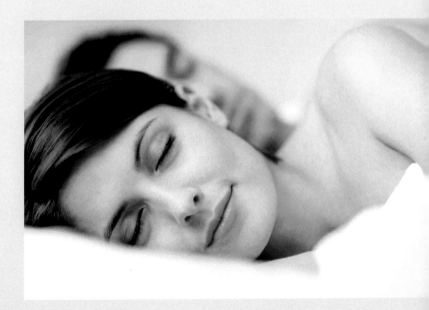

your body's ability to process carbohydrates, which can lead to elevated blood-sugar levels and an increased tendency to store calories as fat. This happens because when you're sleep deprived, your body produces more of the stress hormone cortisol, which seems to set this chain reaction in motion. In other words, loss of sleep can be just as bad for your health as no exercise or a poor diet. Put another way, too little sleep makes you hungry, especially for calorie-dense foods that are not good for you (such as processed carbohydrates and high fatty foods) and primes your body to hold on to the calories you eat.

10 **Nourish your spirit.** To maintain a healthy body, you must first nourish your spirit. The real epidemic in our culture is spiritual heart disease—the experience of low self-esteem combined with feelings of loneliness, isolation and alienation that pervade our culture as I write about in my books *Walking on Air: Your 30-Day Inside and Out Rejuvenation Makeover* and *The Joy Factor: 10 Sacred Practices for Radiant Health*. Many people who suffer from spiritual malaise use food or stimulants such as drugs, caffeine, alcohol, sex or overwork to numb the pain and get through the day.

Stretching, deep breathing and meditation will relax your mind and you will experience a greater sense of peace and well-being. Then you'll be able to make eating and exercise decisions—and other lifestyle choices—that are life-enhancing rather than self-destructive. Engage in physical activities that nourish your body

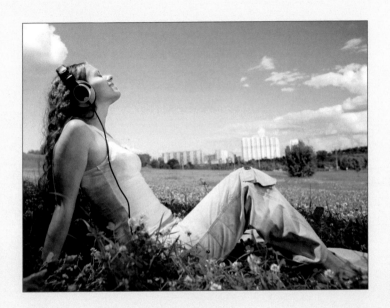

and soul. Cherished activities I enjoy include hiking, gardening, walking at the beach or in a botanical or flower garden, or stretching or yoga (without being in a hurry).

So, in conclusion, dieting alone doesn't work. Good nutrition combined with regular aerobic exercise is better, but it won't replace the muscle tissue that's lost in aging. It's when you combine strength training, aerobic exercise, sensible eating, stress management, meditation and other nourishment for your spirit that you have an unbeatable combination for reaching and maintaining your ideal weight, improving your metabolism, creating a fit, lean body and celebrating life.

Sometimes customizing is necessary because of an injury or the inability to do, for a short or long period, the kind of exercise you formerly did. When you're used to customizing for fun, doing it under duress won't seem like such an imposition. Either way, experiment until you find activities that make you happy as well as healthy. Choose your exercise using the same criteria you'd apply to choosing a date—that is, attractive to you and able to hold your interest for an hour.

—Victoria Moran

HUMOR TIME

If you are going to try cross-country skiing, start with a small country.

—Unknown

I tried every diet in the book. I tried some that weren't in the book. I tried eating the book. It tasted better than most of the diets.

—Dolly Parton

The only reason I would take up jogging is so I could hear heavy breathing again.

—ERMA BOMBECK

Fitness: if it came in a bottle, everybody would have a great body.

—CHER

Be careful about reading health books. You may die of a misprint.

—MARK TWAIN

My swimsuit told me to go to the gym. But my sweatpants were like, Nah girl, you're good!

—UNKNOWN

If swimming is such a good way to stay in shape, explain whales.

—UNKNOWN

The two biggest sellers in any bookstore are the cookbooks and the diet books. The cookbooks tell you how to prepare the food, and the diet books tell you how not to eat any of it!

—ANDY ROONEY

*I think that making love is
the best form of exercise.*

—CARY GRANT

*I have a personal trainer. She makes
me chase rabbits through the woods
three times a day at a dead run.
Also, she has four legs and a tail.*

—UNKNOWN

*When you're old you feast on your
memories, and if you spend too
much time on exercise, you may
get old and not have many.*

—GARRISON KEILLOR

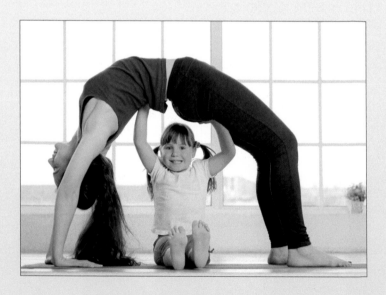

PART 3

Set Up a Positive Magnetic Force

To become master of your outer life, you must first become master of your inner world—CEO of your mind. Teach your mind how to think differently: how to be calm, loving, courageous and optimistic.

—Susan Smith Jones

BEFORE I SHARE WITH YOU SOME OF MY BEST TIPS to staying motivated to exercise and getting positive fitness results without boredom, injury or burnout, I first wanted to shed some light on efficacious ways you can turn your dreams into reality. You have powerful tools within you 24 hours a day; companions that can help you achieve your goals or sabotage you. It's within your power to choose which you implement in your life. Here's what I mean.

Turning Dreams Into Reality

Do you want to live life to the fullest or are you content to just go along with the crowd and settle for whatever comes your way? Your thoughts and beliefs have a strong correlation with every aspect of your life. This is one point upon which brain researchers, physicists, psychologists, psychiatrists, counselors and educators agree. Put simply, you'll get that which you truly believe in and desire.

Take a moment to close your eyes, breathe in deeply and slowly, and scan all the different areas of your life. Is your life a wonderful adventure, filled with celebration and joy? Are your relationships loving and nurturing? Do you enjoy your work and find genuine fulfillment in it? Are you experiencing optimum health and vitality? Is your body lean, strong and finely tuned? More important, are you living a life filled with serenity and peace, sparkling with happiness? If you answered "no" to any of these questions, then this section of the book is written just for you.

Swimming with the Dolphins

A few years ago I had an amazing experience that showed me the tremendous power of thought and bringing your dreams to fruition. I was accustomed to going to the beach in Santa Monica for an invigorating swim a few times each week, very early, and this was a splendid morning just before sunrise. After some stretching exercises and a short run, I was ready for my swim. Because

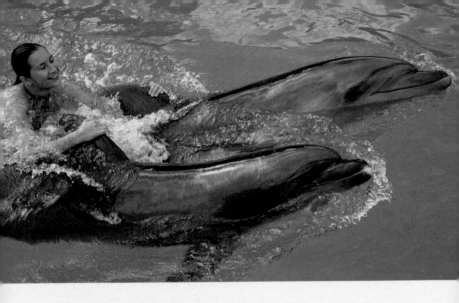

it was the end of summer, the water was still comfortably warm. But this morning there was something in the air that I couldn't quite identify. I felt it deep inside me—a shiver of anticipation, a faint knowing that today would be different, that this day would be one I would remember the rest of my life. I went out into the ocean, rode a few waves and then swam past the swells.

I was aware of the peacefulness of the water. Sparkling and resplendent, it rejuvenated my body and soul with each stroke. A few minutes later some old friends joined me, a group of pelicans who seemed to enjoy escorting me. These marvels of nature have always enthralled me. They were gliding flawlessly a few feet above my head, their wingspan so large that they almost eclipsed the light, when suddenly they flew away. Surprised, I waved good-bye as I turned over to begin the backstroke. It was then I saw something that made my heart plummet.

A large, dark, frightening fin was heading straight for me. Shark! I looked toward the beach. No one was there. I had always taken for granted that I would stay calm in a life-threatening situation. But not this time! As the fin continued in my direction, I simply froze and treaded water. I was so terrified; I couldn't swim away or even cry out. And then it happened—a sight that will forever warm my heart and soul. The fin danced out of the water. It was a dolphin, and it was followed by a school of about two dozen more!

Less than two weeks before, I had watched a television documentary on dolphins. During my meditation that evening, I had visualized myself swimming and playing with a school of dolphins. I accepted and affirmed that that was my desire and reality. I then thanked God for this wonderful experience.

There in the ocean that morning, the dolphins stayed with me for a full half-hour, swimming, jumping out of the water and jumping over me. I swam underwater with them, listening to their mellifluous sounds, touching their skin, feeling a connection and an exchange of love. For what seemed like hours, nothing else existed except my world of dolphins. I was oblivious to any thought of the past or future and lived right in the moment, rejoicing in the thrill of discovery.

Then, as quickly as they had arrived, the dolphins swam off, and I was left alone and immensely grateful. I swam back to shore, where by now a group of people had gathered, captivated by my dance with the dolphins. I answered many questions and tried to share what the experience had been like for me, but I found it very hard to put my feelings into words. Ineffable experiences that speak directly to the heart are often difficult to express clearly.

The others drifted away and I just sat there, enveloped in wonder at the experience of swimming with dolphins, and all I could do was cry—what had happened touched me so lovingly, so profoundly. What a beautiful lesson in living in the present and appreciating each moment. Because of that experience and so many others, I will never doubt the power of thought and belief to create any reality we choose.

Make a Choice

It's time to make a choice. I am going to ask you the same question I mentioned above. Do you want to live life to the fullest, or are you content to just go along with the crowd and settle for whatever comes your way?

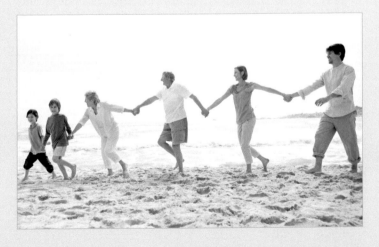

It's always your choice. As Abraham Lincoln so aptly wrote, "We're just about as happy as we make up our minds to be." We adults cannot blame our unhappiness on the environment, our upbringing, our family or friends, our jobs or anything else. We need to take responsibility for ourselves to be all we can be. George Bernard Shaw would probably agree. He said, "People are always blaming their circumstances for what they are. I don't believe in circumstances. The people who get on in this world are the people who get up and look for the circumstances they want and if they can't find them, make them."

In order to become responsible, it is imperative we take a close look at the effect our thoughts and beliefs have on our lives. We each have a conscious mind and a subconscious mind, both of which are responsible for our actions in life. Neither works independently. We are the sum total of all our experiences from the time of our birth until right now.

The conscious mind is the one you use when you analyze, reason and make decisions in your life. The subconscious mind is a storage house for all your experiences, your previous programming and conditioning. The subconscious part of your mind has been influencing your every decision—sometimes in opposition to your conscious desires.

These conflicts occur because the subconscious has little or no reasoning power. It is simply operating like a computer. It functions according to the way it was programmed. In other words, it helps bring into actuality the reality for which it was programmed. Operating like a computer, the subconscious is constantly being fed new programming or data with every thought. Thus you create your own reality with your thoughts, and this reality can be either positive or negative depending on what you are thinking.

All that you have ever dreamed, thought or needed in your life has contributed to what you have at this very moment. So if things aren't just the way you would like them to be, and you want to change them, you must change your thoughts and the words you speak to express those thoughts. Start to reprogram yourself. Andrew Carnegie put it this way, "Any idea that is held in the mind that is either feared or revered will begin at once to clothe itself in the most convenient and appropriate physical forms available."

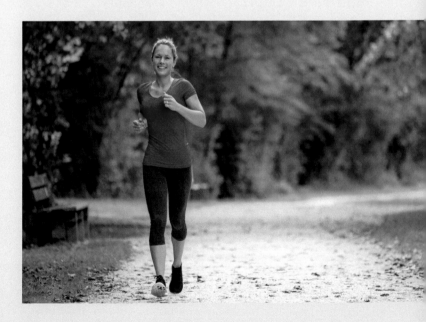

Your Words and Visions
Set Up an Attractive Force

The visions, words and images you hold in your marvelous mind instantly set up a magnetic or attractive force, which governs the experiences in your life. If your image is constantly fluctuating, you will continually be growing into something different, and that sets in motion a most chaotic process. Unfortunately, those individuals who are unaware of these very exact and precise laws are planting images of health, fitness or prosperity in their minds one minute, and then images of the opposite the next. It's very difficult to attract the good in your life when you continually switch from positive to negative thoughts. Strive to keep focused on only those positive things you want to be part of your life.

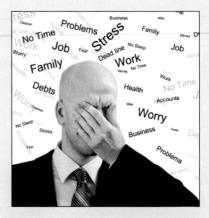

Take a typical day. When you wake up, are you excited and enthusiastic about the new day? Or are you reluctant, preoccupied with the discordant alarm clock, the hurry and traffic on the way to work, job dissatisfaction and dissatisfaction with yourself in general? Those negative thoughts can persist all during the day. And if you think these thoughts don't add up, you'd better think again.

According to the National Science Foundation, you think thousands of thoughts every day—in fact, about 1,000 an hour. The ordinary human being thinks about 12,000 thoughts a day. A deeper thinker (most likely you, of course!), according to this report, generates about 50,000 thoughts. So imagine that 50 percent of the time you are positive in your thoughts. For you, that means 25,000 negative thoughts are being added to your programming every day. And these thoughts are influencing the reality you have created for yourself.

Keep in mind that although the subconscious part of our mind programs us, it doesn't reason and it doesn't have a sense of humor. Rather, it works to create the reality according to the programming it has been fed. This is normally accomplished by thoughts and through your life experiences, but brain researchers have found that since the subconscious is incapable of telling the difference between reality and fantasy, between the real experience and the imagined experience, it also programs your goals, aspirations, beliefs and other attitudes you have about life.

A study at the University of Chicago was done on the relationship of visualization to sports ability. Subjects were divided into three groups and basketball was the sport used in the experiment. At the beginning, all the participants were tested as to their individual basket-shooting ability and the results were recorded. Then Group One was told, "You are each to practice shooting baskets for 20 minutes a day for 20 days." Group Two was told, "Don't play any basketball for 20 days. In fact, just forget about basketball for the entire time." Group Three was told, "You are to spend 20 minutes a day *imagining* you are *successfully* shooting baskets. Do this every day for 20 days. See every detail of your accomplishments in your mind."

At the conclusion, the three groups were tested again. Group Two members, who hadn't played basketball for 20 days, showed no improvement. Group One members, who had been practicing 20 minutes a day for 20 days, showed a 24 percent improvement in their basket-shooting ability. Group Three members, who had only *imagined* that they 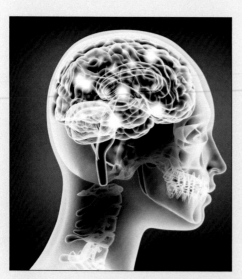 were *successfully* shooting baskets for 20 minutes a day, showed a 23 percent improvement in their actual basket-shooting ability—*only one percentage point less* than the group that had actually been practicing! That's so astounding, profound and enlightening to me.

The subconscious can be programmed to procure the results you desire. With this knowledge, you can work on any area of your life. Here are some practical steps you can take.

The Magic of Creative Visualization

A couple of times a day, especially when you wake up in the morning and just before you go to sleep at night, create some mental movies (creative visualization) that star yourself. Be as specific and precise as you can. For example, if you are working in an area that involves other people, include them in your movie. Use your imagination and visualize all the details you can.

See yourself behaving exactly as you wish to behave in real life. Experience it, enjoy it and see it just the way you would like it to be. See yourself relaxed, confident and feeling positive about you. Go through the entire movie and, when you get to the end, experience how wonderful it *feels* to have behaved in such a positive manner.

The key is to see and experience only the way you would like it to be—*successful* and *positive*. You can choose to work on one goal at a time or several goals. It's up to you. It's also best to combine the visualizations with positive affirmations, as you'll learn about below.

This is the kind of positive programming I teach my clients in my lectures and workshops around the world to use for every area of their lives—from their level of fitness, to their overall health, to their relationships, job satisfaction, level of wealth and prosperity, and balanced lifestyle.

Let me emphasize that this type of programming doesn't take the place of the practice time required to learn new habits or develop new skills. But it does add two new ingredients—commitment and enjoyment—to everyday living.

Before we move on to Part 4, I wanted to share with you another personal story that happened in my life that highlights the power of our thoughts, visualization, hopes and positive expectations.

My First Marathon Race Experience

I don't think this was simply a random happening. See what you think. In the '70s, I ran my first marathon in December in Culver City (in the Los Angeles area). I had devoted a year to training. When the race day arrived, my emotions were mixed. On the one hand, I was eager and excited to run, although not quite sure what to expect since I had never done this before. On the other hand, I was feeling sad. The day of the race was the one-year anniversary of my grandmother Fritzie's death. Fritzie had been instrumental in teaching me about my own spirituality, about self-reliance, simplicity and living fully. As I was driving to Culver City the morning of the race, I felt a tremendous longing to visit with her; I missed her so much. In the car, I was actually talking with her out loud as a way to soothe my heart. I even said to her that I was open to her spirit and energy. I asked her to let me know somehow if she could hear me and to please help me through the marathon.

When I arrived at the race site, there were lots of

people getting ready. I was wishing I knew someone so I wouldn't have to run alone. The gun went off and so did several thousand runners. For the first three miles, I was alone and felt great—confident, relaxed and energetic. Around the fourth mile, a young man who looked to be in his mid-twenties ran up next to me and we began talking. Before we knew it, we were at mile ten, then fifteen, then twenty. It's amazing the things you'll tell someone you've never met when you're running together. I think it has something to do with the release of certain chemicals in the body and a change in the electrical activity of the brain during aerobic activity. We talked about our lives, families, interests, dreams and goals. I was feeling extremely grateful to him because our conversation made the miles sail by.

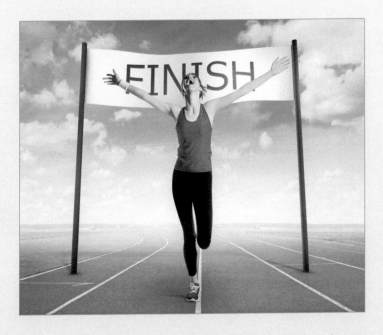

Before we knew it, we were at mile twenty-five. At this point in our conversation, we started talking about where we lived. I told him I lived in Brentwood and he told me he lived in Studio City. "That's interesting," I said. "My grandmother used to live in Studio City. What street do you live on?" When he told me the street, I gasped, for it was the same street as Fritzie. At this point, we were close to the finish line. I had just enough time to inquire about his exact location. We were crossing the finish line when he told me he had moved into his home eleven months earlier, and that the lady who lived there before him had passed away. I could hardly breathe, not because I was tired, but because of what he was telling me. He had moved into Fritzie's house!

Coincidence you say? I don't think so. Out of all the thousands of people in the race, how did I end up running with the man who lived in my grandmother's home? And how do you explain this happening only a few hours after I had asked Fritzie to give me some sign that she was receiving my communication?

Only believe. Have faith. Trust your inner guidance. Fill your imagination with those things you want to create in your life. Support these visualizations with positive words, positive expectations and feelings of gratitude that this is your current reality—because it is already on another level. The world is yours for the asking. It was Albert Einstein who once said: *Your imagination is a preview of your life's coming attractions.* And he was a very smart man.

A feeble body weakens the mind.

—Jean-Jacques Rousseau

HUMOR  TIME

*I'm opening a gym called "Resolutions."
It will have exercise equipment for
the first two weeks and then turn
into a bar for the rest of the year!*

—Unknown

*I was wondering today why brain cells
die, skin cells die, and hair follicles
die, but fat cells live FOREVER!*

—Unknown

*One of the hardest meals for me
to limit myself is the one from
Halloween till New Years.*

—Unknown

*If you think a minute goes by really
fast, you've never been on a treadmill.*

—Unknown

I tried exercise but found I was allergic to it—my skin flushed, my heart raced, I got sweaty, short of breath. Very, very dangerous.

—Unknown

I believe that every human has a finite amount of heartbeats. I don't intend to waste any of mine running around doing exercises.

—Neil Armstrong

Got up to 40 minutes on the exercise bike! Next week I'm going to try turning the pedals.

—Unknown

It's funny how exercise helps you live longer because whenever I exercise, it makes me feel like I'm dying.

—Unknown

An onion can make people cry but there's never a vegetable that can make people laugh.

—Will Rogers

PART 4

Surefire Tips to Enjoy, Enrich & Energize Your Workouts

I think exercise tests us in so many ways, our skills, our hearts, our ability to bounce back after setbacks. This is the inner beauty of sports and competition, and it can serve us all well as adult athletes.

—PEGGY FLEMING

THERE'S NO DOUBT ABOUT IT. EVERY PERSON WHO exercises regularly, whether an athlete or not, will have to cope with lack of enthusiasm at one time or another. So how can you stay motivated to workout? "Just do it" was one of Nike's rallying slogans of the late '90s. But sometimes it can be tough to live up to. In fact, every person who decides to exercise will face—sooner or later—a lack of motivation, boredom, or burnout with a fitness program.

So at this point in the book, my wish is that you are now ready to embark on a regular fitness program and give it your all. Here are a few of my best tips to help you stay motivated, prevent injury and preclude burnout and boredom. You will find more comprehensive information on how to stay motivated, lose weight, feel happy, attract unlimited abundance, disease-proof your body and create your best life in my books and on my website—**www.SusanSmithJones.com**.

1 Make a commitment. To succeed in anything in life, especially in your exercise goals, you must be committed. I often hear people tell me they're really committed to their exercise program, but they can't exercise for a week or two because they're too busy.

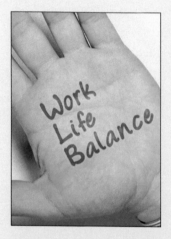 When you're committed to something, you don't let your excuses get in the way. And if you are ready for commitment, you will be committed; you'll immediately arrange your personal circumstances so that your lifestyle totally supports your commitment. You will do the things you need to do to order your life, eliminate non-essentials, and focus on what is important. If you have a difficult time sticking with your exercise program, keep in mind that you should be working out because you want to do it for you and not because you are doing it to please someone else. Others can provide some incentive, but the prime reason must come

from your own desire. Practice being disciplined. I see *discipline as the ability to carry out a resolution long after the mood and enthusiasm have left you.*

You will be successful. Believe in yourself and stick with your commitment. It was Will Rogers who said this: "If you want to be successful, it's just this simple. Know what you are doing. Love what you are doing. And believe in what you are doing."

2 **Be consistent.** Repetition is the key to mastery—lack of it is the road to failure. Behavioral scientists have discovered that it takes at least 21 days for your mind and body to create a new habit and to stop resisting. Until then, you can expect to have to listen to that incessant voice in the back of your mind. I call that voice "Babbler," because it never shuts up. You

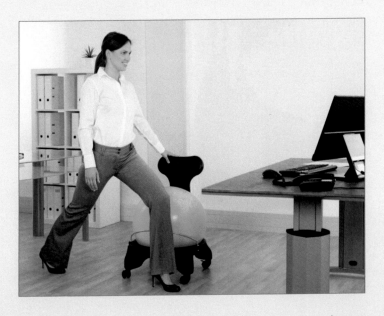

can count on Babbler to keep up a running dialogue on how nice it would be to sleep in, how sore your calf muscles are or how heavy the weights feel. Don't pay any attention. Instead, when the commentary begins, simply acknowledge Babbler's point of view and remind yourself that for 21 *consecutive* days you are going to stick to your new exercise program. By the end of the 21-day period, chances are you'll no longer have any resistance to exercising. Ben Franklin once said that whatever you do for 21 days will make or break a habit. And he's right.

Make a 21-day agreement with yourself, an investment in *yourself,* to exercise. In the Search Bar of my website, **www.SusanSmithJones.com**, put in the words *21-Day Agreement,* and you will find a one-page form that you can print out to use for your agreements to help keep you on track. Also, you'll find more detailed information on how to use 21-day agreements to help you achieve your goals in record-breaking time.

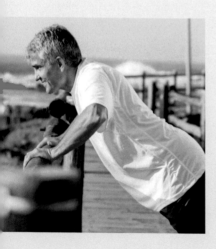

In my website's Search Bar, also type in *Push-Away: A Strength-Building Exercise for Everyone.* This is a simple exercise that I recommend you do daily. This would be an excellent 21-day agreement to do *Push-Aways* every day in the beginning, intermediate or advanced forms as taught on my website.

3 **Clearly define your fitness goals.** Make both short- and long-term goals. Short-term goals are important because with them you become immediately involved with the life process. Since short-term goals are usually fairly easy to reach, you receive early reinforcement of your intentions. You are rewarded for positive action and this creates a positive mental attitude, builds confidence and tends to neutralize failure patterns imprinted in the subconscious.

Yes, goals provide a path for specific direction and also let you know how you are doing. What are your goals for exercising and being fit? To lose weight and reshape your body? To increase your energy and boost your self-esteem? Perhaps you want to be able to run in a 10K race or increase your strength and definition? Whatever is important to you, write it down on paper. Just because goals are on paper doesn't mean they can't be changed at some point.

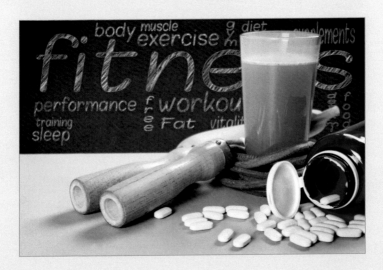

4 **Reaffirm your fitness goals daily.** After you've written your fitness goals, post them where you can see them every day—perhaps on the refrigerator door or on the bathroom mirror. As you achieve your goals, set new ones. In addition to a concise list of goals, make another list of your plan for achieving your goals. Let's say that you've been jogging for six months and you're now up to four miles, four times a week. One of your goals is to run a 10K race in a month, a marathon a year from now, and to increase your strength and

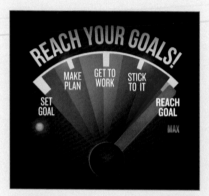

lose inches by lifting weights. You'd then map out a jogging program that gradually increases your mileage weekly in addition to working on a specific weight-training program to suit your needs. This is the procedure I followed when training to run 100 miles from Santa Barbara to Los Angeles and training for seven marathons and several triathlons, as well as when I decide to lose a few pounds or want to increase strength or flexibility.

5 **Keep track of your daily progress.** In one of the rooms of my home, I've displayed on the wall a large year-at-a-glance calendar on which I can write my workouts everyday. For me, this is highly motivating to see all that I've accomplished over the past

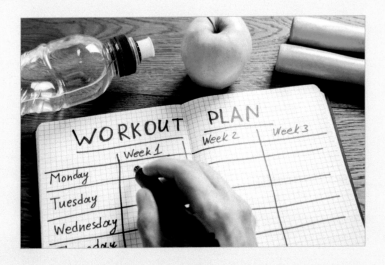

weeks and months of training. On those days when I lack motivation to work out, I look at the calendar and realize I don't want to ruin my track record with too many non-workout days. You may also want to consider keeping a fitness diary.

6 Share your fitness goals with a friend. I have always found it beneficial to confide in a friend(s) and tell them my goals. Oftentimes it's easy to let yourself down and break commitments, but it's harder to get off the course when a caring, supportive friend is checking up to see how you're progressing. But make sure it's a trusted

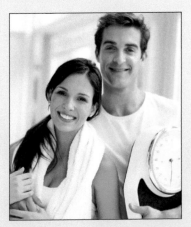

friend with whom you feel comfortable and not someone who will bring up your "slip backs" (and you will have some!) at the next office party.

7 **Be realistic.** Don't set yourself up to fail. If you've just started a walking program and are now up to two miles nonstop, don't make one of your goals to run a marathon at the end of the month. I'm not suggesting that it's impossible. I believe in miracles, but it would definitely take a miracle for a typical person to get in shape for a marathon that quickly and part of staying motivated to exercise is staying injury-free.

Setting your goals will help you to be realistic. Make three lists of goals: one to cover the next month (these can be changed daily or weekly), one for the next six months (these might change monthly), and one to cover the entire year (these might change quarterly).

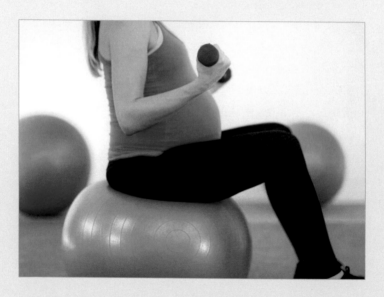

8 **Exercise with a friend.** It can sometimes be easier when you have a friend to give you support. As mentioned above, it's harder to let a friend down when you've agreed to work out together. I enjoy training alone at times, but many times I'm grateful to friends for getting me through workouts I probably would have skipped if I were working out alone. Working out with a friend helps to prevent boredom. My closest friendships throughout my life have been with those friends with whom I workout on a regular basis.

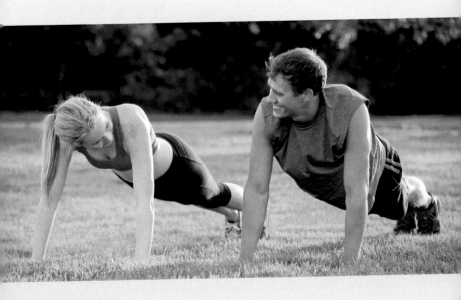

9 **Listen to music or nature while exercising.** Music can work wonders, either through a radio, headphones, or just singing, if the activity is adaptable to it. I have a home gym and find that my favorite music keeps me motivated especially when lifting weights or

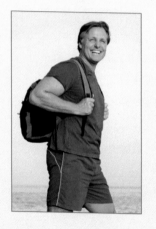

using the treadmill or rower. When I'm hiking outdoors in the mountains, my favorite music comes from nature—the songs of the birds, the breeze wafting through the trees, the creek or river flowing aplenty, the sound of the hummingbird wings and much more.

10 **Keep variety in your workouts.** To keep exercise interesting—and lower the likelihood of injury—alternate high-impact activities like step aerobics, spinning, jogging or hiking steep hills with low-impact ones such as Pilates, yoga, swimming or walking. Vary your activities, known as cross-training, so that you won't get bored and will ensure a more balanced body fitness. And make sure you select accessible activities. Go to a nearby aerobics class or health club, swim in your pool or local university or community pool. Have a few pieces of equipment in your home for those days you can't get away to work out.

Remember, whenever possible, exercise outdoors in nature. One of my favorite ways to exercise, as you read about in Part 1, is hiking. It works out my body and rejuvenates my mind and soul. And I also like to ride horses. It's an excellent way to stimulate hundreds of muscles, ligaments and tendons in your body and, like hiking or walking/jogging at the beach, it also feeds your soul.

11 **Visualize your fitness goals.** As mentioned already in Part 3 of this book, visualizing your fitness goals as already accomplished will increase your motivation, keep you on course and hasten your success. Remember, the subconscious part of the brain cannot tell the difference between fantasy and reality, between the visualization and the actual event taking place. In doing this on a regular basis, you will discover that your actions and behavior regarding the achievement of your goal seem to come into alignment more easily and readily, without as much resistance, and you continue in the right direction sometimes achieving goals in unexpected time.

I love what Henry David Thoreau once said. "If you advance confidently in the direction of your dreams and endeavor to live the life you have imagined, you will meet with a success unexpected in common hours." He also said, "An early morning walk is a blessing for the whole day."

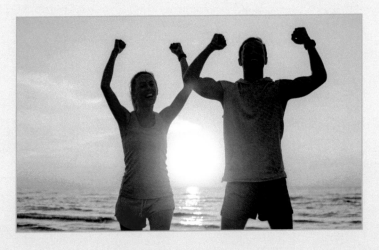

12 Use affirmations to support your goals.

This tool greatly enhances motivation. Affirmations can be mental, verbal, written or recorded and played back on a CD or other listening device like an iPod. An affirmation is the result of a purposeful effort to synchronize thought, speech and feeling in order to produce definite effects. An affirmation, used properly, is not a drill used to condition the mind; it is a technique that gives us conscious control over thought and attitude. Select a phrase that embodies your idea; again, working from the end of the idealized condition. When you synchronize your thoughts, words and feelings, you become magnetized and your power of concentration is focused on specific targets, or goals. For example, you might affirm the following: *"I am fit, healthy, and at my ideal weight of (fill in the blank); I enjoy my workouts and keep my word to exercise at least four times a week."* (See another affirmation below.)

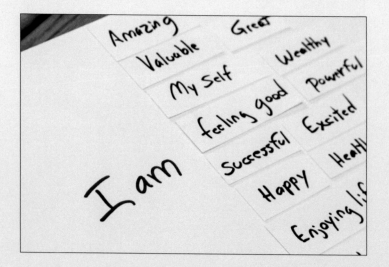

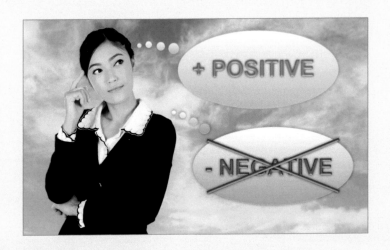

13 **Stay positive and present.** When using affirmations, it's important to remember the following: Always keep the affirmation in the present tense, as though this were your present reality. Also, keep the affirmation positive. For instance, you might use a phrase like, *"I am now healthy, fit and filled with energy and enthusiasm for life. My body is strong, trim and beautifully shaped. I choose only those foods that support my health and continual rejuvenation. I exercise on a regular basis and am delighted with how good I look and feel."*

Keep positive and present. For example, instead of saying, *"I will never eat junk food again and am not fat,"* say, *"I select healthy foods that support my trim, fit body."*

And finally, use your affirmations with feeling. Experience the joy, enthusiasm and positive feeling you would really have if this affirmation were your current reality. Practice using your affirmations daily, especially right before you go to sleep at night and upon awakening in the morning.

14 **Rest one day per week.** After your initial 21-day period of daily exercise to establish a new habit, take one day a week off for rest each week. Maybe on those rest days you will stretch, do some yoga or easy walking. Taking a day off allows the body to repair the muscles and build up more energy. This also helps to avoid injury from overuse. Taking some time off is also great for keeping your motivation up. Don't feel guilty. Weekly respites from exercise are good for your body.

15 **Exercise outdoors.** New research from England's University of Essex discloses that just five minutes of "green exercise" such as skating, walking in the park or around your neighborhood, gardening, biking, hiking, etc., can boost your self-esteem and mood. This study is consistent with previous research showing that outdoor walks combat depression much better than mall walks do. Also, if you exercise outdoors, chances are that you'll get more exposure to health-promoting vitamin D (from the sun) and could be spending less time in the doctor's office. Among other things, getting ample vitamin D brightens your mood and helps you see things in a more positive light. As I tell my clients in my private practice, my friends and family, take your workouts outdoors in nature, if you want to fix what ails you and stay motivated to stick with your program. Being in nature is one of the best ways to heal and rejuvenate your body, mind and spirit.

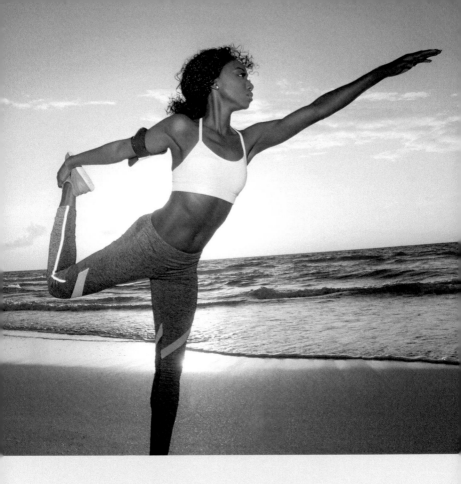

Find new places to walk your dog(s) out in nature, too. Just as you would get tired of doing the same, familiar walk around your neighborhood everyday for months, your beloved dogs also need adventures and appreciate exciting, new scenery, too, especially out in nature. And as you are getting in shape, so will your dog. Be sure to step up the pace, when possible, so both of you get a great cardio workout. Whenever possible, find hills to climb with expansive views to feed your body and soul (as you see on this book's cover).

16 **Reward yourself.** You've worked out hard, you've been consistent and you're seeing positive changes in your body, so go ahead and reward yourself. Enjoy a trigger point massage, buy yourself new exercise clothes or shoes, or take a few hours off just for you to be pampered or simply spend time alone out in nature. Treat yourself to something special because you deserve it! Rewards increase motivation and create positive, happy associations about your exercise program.

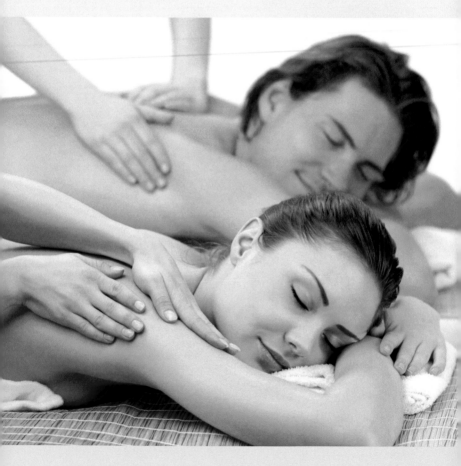

No one is going to be highly motivated to work out 100 percent of the time, but if you follow the guidelines suggested above, you will keep your exercise burnout, boredom or injury to a minimum. For those of you who have an exercise program and are rarely motivated or lack consistency, think about the following: Is it lack of variety? An emotional challenge? What are you afraid of if you achieve your fitness goals? Are you pushing too hard? Do you have clear-cut short- and long-term fitness goals? Have you decided that getting in better shape is not a top priority for you? Keep in mind that you should be working out because you want to do it for you and not because you are doing it to please someone else.

Today, commit to your exercise program. Accept and expect the best for yourself and advance confidently in the direction of your goals and dreams. I believe in you and know you can achieve your goals and dreams to be a fit, healthy, prosperous, successful and balanced being!

After you've made progress with your fitness goals and want something new to implement into your exercise program, how about this? For those of you who feel so inclined to do something very special that will enrich and enhance your life immeasurably, I will end this book with my final section on *How Prayer-Walking & Prayer-Hiking Can Enrich Your Life—Physically, Emotionally, Mentally & Spiritually.*

HUMOR  TIME

When I exercise, I wear all black.
It's like a funeral for my fat.

—UNKNOWN

I really don't think I need buns of steel.
I'd be happier with buns of cinnamon.

—ELLEN DeGENERES

I do two hours of cardio every
day. But I still need to find the
closest parking spot to the gym.

—UNKNOWN

Laugh . . . and the world laughs
with you. Go to the gym at 4:00
in the morning . . . and you've
got the whole gym to yourself!

—UNKNOWN

Someone call CSI.
I just killed my workout.

—UNKNOWN

My idea of exercise is a good, brisk sit.

—Phyllis Diller

*I forgot to post on Facebook I was
going to the gym. Now this whole
workout was a waste of time.*

—Unknown

*No time for to go to the gym?
Please tell me how you watch
three hours of TV every night.*

—Unknown

*Don't you hate it when you're doing
push-ups and you lose
count after 1,000?*

—Unknown

*Whenever I feel the need to exercise,
I lie down until it goes away.*

—Robert Maynard Hutchins

*America has got to be the only country
in the world where people need energy
drinks to sit in front of a computer.*

—Unknown

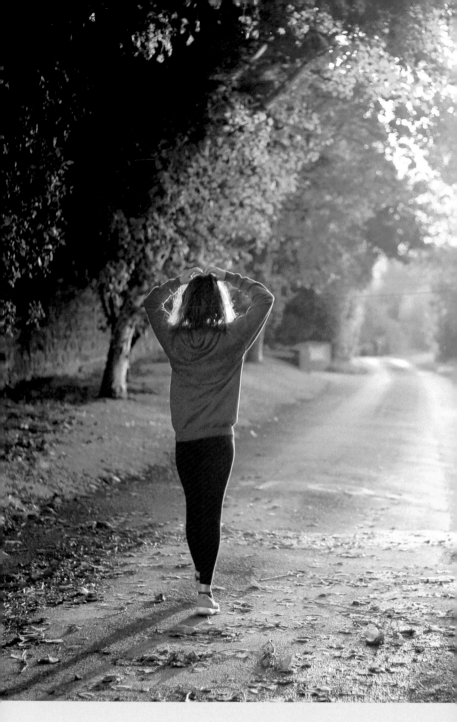

How Prayer-Walking & Prayer-Hiking Can Enrich Your Life— Physically, Emotionally, Mentally & Spiritually

Obviously, your family life is the priority, but there's still other stuff you have to get done in a day. I think the way I make it work is by taking care of myself, and that includes fitness and eating right and all those things, but also being very organized and punctual.

—CINDY CRAWFORD

I'VE BEEN DOING PRAYER-WALKS AND PRAYER-HIKES for three decades. I find it a winning combination that improves my health and well-being and nourishes my mind and soul at the same time. For those of you who are into multitasking and making good use of your oh-so-limited time, this concept of combining walking and prayer should be most appealing.

Most of us are busy talking all day long. Just 20 minutes of walking in silent contemplation can slow down the mind, relax the body and feed the soul. Besides, it's a practical and efficient way to preclude overloading the daily schedule!

When I teach this kind of walking, I tell beginners to start with 20 minutes at least three times a week. Make sure to walk fast enough to elevate your heart rate so that you will get a workout. Of course, if you're not a beginner, you can walk longer for more benefits. On days when, for whatever reason, you don't feel like walking fast, it's all right to go at a more leisurely pace.

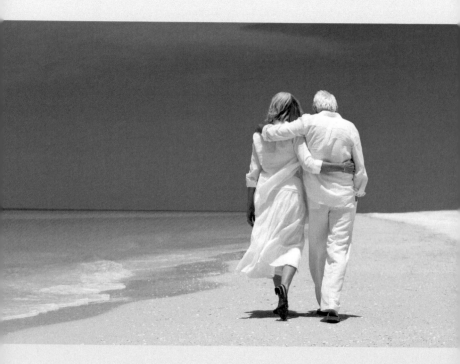

Best Locations to Do Prayer-Walking

When I do prayer-walking; I select places in nature, whether in the mountains, by the ocean, in the desert, or at a botanical garden or local park. I try to find areas with the least noise and the fewest people, especially places where I won't run into anyone I know. It can be very disconcerting, when you've been prayer-walking for 20 or 30 minutes and are deeply into your inner reflection, to hear someone call your name and come over for a chat. If that happens, politely say that you're doing a special silent workout today and will be happy to give them a call later on. That usually works. If not, enjoy the encounter and then pick up where you left off, or try again another day.

What I've learned about prayer-walking is even truer of prayer-hiking. Prayer-hiking is the ultimate experience for me because I'm enveloped in the musical sounds of nature, the majesty of the trees, the fresh air, the fragrance of the surroundings and the subtle whisperings of the angelic forces all around. When I make my hike a prayer-hike, I choose paths I know well so that my mind won't deviate from its inner focus to figure out which way to go. Since I've hiked the Santa Monica Mountains for over three decades, and now some trails throughout Great Britain for years, I know the idiosyncrasies and nuances of all the different trails very well. You can conduct a prayer-hike with a friend or two, knowing that you'll choose silence during the hike and catch up on things when the hike

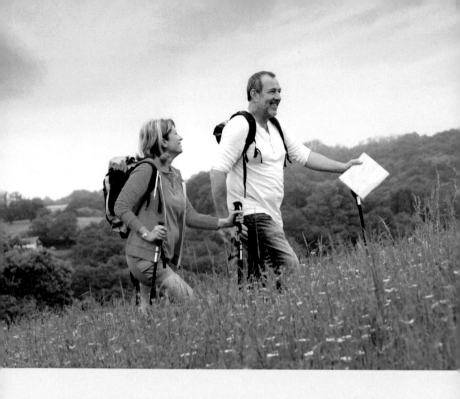

is over. If you can't resist conversation when a friend is around, however, you might choose to prayer-hike alone in order to garner the most benefits for body, mind, and spirit.

Turn on any news program or read any newspaper and you'll doubtless find information abounding on crime, terrorism, violence, war and every kind of abuse. The information alone is enough to create within us fear, frustration, confusion and disharmony. The most effective way I know to restore balance and foster serenity is to appreciate beauty. Of course you can visit a museum, listen to a symphony, watch an awe-inspiring movie or arrange some freshly cut flowers in your home, but I think simply being out in nature is the best. The natural environment is the most fundamental form of beauty, and it's absolutely free. When you are "out of sorts" and need to be reconnected with your own true beauty and best self, nature will gently steer you in the right direction. Our hearts and minds resonate with the amazing colors and sounds of nature, and our cells actually begin to vibrate at a higher frequency that affords a deeper spiritual connection and a feeling of belonging.

Prayer-Walking and Hiking for Life-Enriching Mental and Spiritual Discipline

By silently communing with what is around us, we can learn many things, and this is especially true when it comes to prayer-hiking. Sometimes, instead of repeating an affirmation or mantra, I will simply stay in the present during the hike, breathe deeply and focus on and appreciate the beauty all around me. This is much harder to do than you might think. When I first started doing it, my mind seemed to wander every few seconds like an untrained puppy, to every subject but the task at hand—appreciating the beauty of my surroundings.

It took about a year, prayer-hiking four to six times monthly, for me to be able to do an entire one- or two-hour hike absorbed in nothing but the present and the beauty around me. Like anything worth learning, prayerhiking takes disciplined practice, but the effort has made a positive, profound difference in all areas of my life. The physical and mental discipline brings spiritual discipline, and when all three are in harmony, all directed by the same desire and intention, I feel faith-filled, empowered and invincible.

And, most important to me, I feel divinely guided and loved by God and connected to everything good and loving. And so will you!

I salute your commitment to exercise and great adventure of living fully, and I hope to meet you somewhere along the path of life.

Cheers,

Susan

Susan Smith Jones, PhD

Reading is to the mind what exercise is to the body; they stimulate, rejuvenate and empower the individual.
—SUSAN SMITH JONES

More Inspirational Quotes for Encouragement

I only went out for a walk and finally concluded to stay out till sundown, for going out, I found, was really going in.

—JOHN MUIR

A man may take as much exercise in walking a mile up and down stairs, as in ten on level ground.

—BENJAMIN FRANKLIN

Lack of activity destroys the good condition of every human being, while movement and methodical physical exercise save it and preserve it.

—PLATO

Champions aren't made in the gyms. Champions are made from something they have deep inside them—a desire, a dream, a vision.

—MUHAMMAD ALI

*I feel better in my mind when I work
out. It makes everything better.*
—KERI RUSSELL

The secret of getting ahead is getting started.
—MARK TWAIN

Don't wait. The time will never be just right.
—NAPOLEON HILL

*Physical fitness can neither be achieved by
wishful thinking nor outright purchase.*
—JOSEPH PILATES

*Nothing great was ever achieved
without enthusiasm.*
—RALPH WALDO EMERSON

*Me thinks that the moment my legs begin
to move, my thoughts begin to flow.*
—HENRY DAVID THOREAU

You must do the thing you think you cannot do.
—ELEANOR ROOSEVELT

*You may be disappointed if you fail,
but you are doomed if you do not try.*
—BEVERLY SILLS

Definition of Success

by Ralph Waldo Emerson

To laugh often and much,
to win respect of intelligent people
and the affection of children;
to earn the appreciation of honest critics
and endure the betrayal of false friends;
to appreciate beauty;
to find the best in others;
to leave the world a bit better
whether by a healthy child,
a garden patch, or a
redeemed social condition;
to know even one life
has breathed easier
because you have lived.
This is to have succeeded.

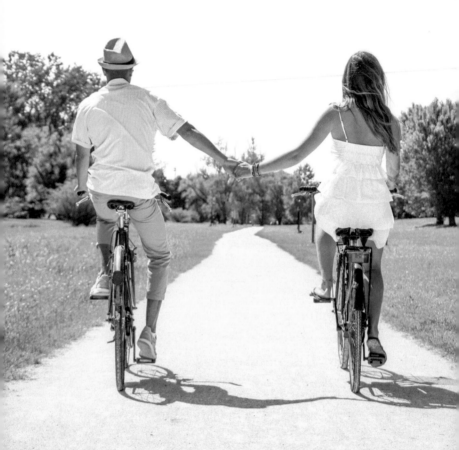

Resources

Please refer to **www.SusanSmithJones.com** to learn more about, or to purchase, these books. You will find the full list of Susan's titles on her website.

The Joy Factor

Health Bliss

The Healing Power of NatureFoods

Recipes for Health Bliss

Conquer Colds & Allergies

The Curative Kitchen & Lifestyle

Healthy, Happy & Radiant . . . at Any Age

Living on the Lighter Side

Discover the Healing Secrets in Your Spice Rack

Nature's Medicine Chest

Choose to Live Peacefully

Wired to Meditate

Walking on Air

Vegetable Soup/The Fruit Bowl
(co-authored with Dianne Warren)

If you'd like to receive Susan's free monthly *Healthy Living Newsletters* filled with uplifting, empowering and high-powered information, go to her website's Search Bar and type in the words *Subscribe & Win!* It takes only 15 seconds to sign-up and you will also receive several gifts from Susan.

About
Susan Smith Jones, PhD

*Any idea that is held in the mind
that is either feared or revered will
begin at once to clothe itself in the
most convenient and appropriate
physical forms available.*

—ANDREW CARNEGIE

For a woman with three of America's and the UK's most ordinary names, **Dr. Susan Smith Jones** has certainly made extraordinary contributions in the fields of holistic health, longevity, optimum nutrition, high-level fitness and balanced, peaceful living. For starters, she taught students, staff and faculty at UCLA how to be healthy and fit for 30 years!

Susan is the founder and president of Health Unlimited, a Los Angeles-based consulting firm dedicated to optimal wellness and holistic health education. As a renowned motivational speaker, Susan

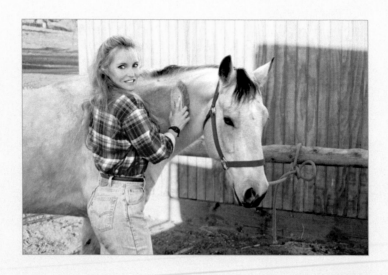

travels internationally as a frequent radio/TV talk show guest and motivational speaker (seminars, workshops, lectures and keynote address); she's also the author of more than 2,000 magazine articles and over 25 books, including—*The Curative Kitchen & Lifestyle; Living on the Lighter Side; Healthy, Happy & Radiant . . . at Any Age; Recipes for Health Bliss; The Healing Power of NatureFoods; Health Bliss; Walking on Air: Your 30-Day, Inside and Out Rejuvenation Makeover;* and *The Joy Factor: 10 Sacred Practices for Radiant Health.*

Susan is in a unique position to testify on the efficacy of her basic message that health is the result of choice. When her back was fractured in an automobile accident, her physician told her that she would never be able to carry "anything heavier than a small purse." Susan chose not to accept this verdict; within six months, there was no longer any pain or evidence of the fracture. Soon, she fully regained her health and active lifestyle. Susan attributes her healing to her natural-foods diet, a daily well-rounded fitness program, the power of Spirit, faith, determination, balanced living and a deep commitment to expressing her highest potential. Since that time, she has been constantly active in spreading the message that anyone can choose radiant health and rejuvenation. Her inspiring message and innovative techniques for achieving total health in body, mind and spirit have won her a grateful and enthusiastic following and have put her in constant demand internationally as a health and fitness consultant and educator. A gifted teacher, Susan brings together modern research and ageless wisdom in all of her work. When she's not traveling the world, she resides in both West Los Angeles and England.

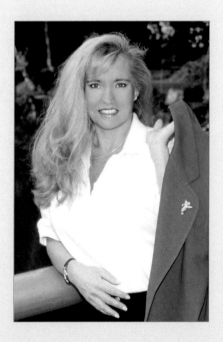

For more details on Susan and her work, please visit: **www.SusanSmithJones.com**. Susan's books and website are like having a **"holistic health app"** for anything health-related. Her website is a cornucopia of articles, photos and the latest information you won't want to be without on superfoods, optimal nutrition, easy weight loss, high-level fitness, longevity, rejuvenation, detoxification, meditation, spiritual health, natural remedies and balanced living.

People are always blaming their circumstances for what they are. I don't believe in circumstances. The people who get on in this world are the people who get up and look for the circumstances they want and if they can't find them, make them.

—George Bernard Shaw

NOTES

NOTES